An Atlas of Glass-Ionomer Cements:

A Clinician's Guide

Clinical Techniques in Dentistry

An Atlas of Glass-Ionomer Cements:

A Clinician's Guide

Graham J Mount, AM

BDS, FRACDS, FICD, FADI

MARTIN DUNITZ

Cover illustrations

Above: Class V erosion lesions in three teeth, 5 years after restoration with glass-ionomer cement. No cavity preparation was carried out. The cement was handled correctly and allowed to mature fully.

Centre: Erosion lesions on the labial of both upper central incisors, 2 years after restoration with glass-ionomer cement alone.

Below: An upper right first molar with an extensive erosion lesion restored with glass-ionomer cement. This photograph was taken 2 years after placement.

© **Graham J Mount 1990**

First published in the United Kingdom in 1990 by
Martin Dunitz Ltd, 154 Camden High Street, London NW1 0NE

British Library Cataloguing in Publication Data

Mount, Graham J.
  An atlas of glass-ionomer cements.
  1. Dental materials
  I. Title
  617.6'95
  ISBN 1–85317–006–2

Laserset by Scribe Design, Gillingham, Kent
Colour origination by Imago Publishing Ltd
Manufactured by Imago Publishing Ltd
Printed and bound in Hong Kong

Contents

Foreword

The invention of the glass-ionomer cement in 1969 (first reported by Wilson and Kent in 1971) resulted from a programme of work at the Laboratory of The Government Chemist to eliminate some of the deficiencies in the dental silicate cements. I was privileged to participate in this programme and subsequently to introduce the first glass-ionomer cements to the dental profession. It need hardly be said that the path ahead proved to be a stony one. This experience was shared by FN Doubleday in 1920 when he was referring to his investigations into translucent filling cements. He quoted the first medical aphorism by Hippocrates, 'Life is short, art long, opportunity fleeting, experiment slippery, judgment difficult' and added, 'He who attempts to investigate translucent cement fillings learns by experience its truth'. I certainly did. However, despite the early shortcomings of the original ASPA glass-ionomer cement, it is interesting to note that restorations in this material are still surviving after 14 years in service. Indeed, providing the cement was adequately protected with varnish in its early setting stage, the physical properties of ASPA have only recently been surpassed. Snap judgments on new materials and ill-conceived in vitro experiments can often lead to the demise of a new system which may have the potential to make a significant contribution to public health. Fortunately this did not occur with the glass-ionomer cements and Dr Mount should take much of the credit for this.

My first contact with Graham Mount was at the Australian Congress in Adelaide in 1976. I met a kindred spirit who quickly recognized the enormous potential in this new hydrophilic material, the major assets being long-term adhesion to tooth structure, minimal shrinkage and low thermal expansion, and perhaps more importantly a cariostatic property due to the ability of the cement to leach fluoride. It is only recently that the profession has recognized the advantages of treating early dental caries with glass-ionomer cements. Graham Mount has pioneered much of this work and it clearly shows in his writing. The use of micro-cutting techniques is now mandatory for the treatment of early dental caries and glass-ionomer lining cements are becoming increasingly popular for attaching composites to dentine. The silver-reinforced cement-ionomer cements play a growing role in the treatment of the geriatric patient and in the restoration of the Class II lesion via an internal occlusal fossa or 'tunnel' preparation.

Dr Mount's atlas offers the general practitioner the opportunity to familiarize himself quickly with this new technology, since the illustrations are backed up by a wealth of clinical experience gained over many years. I hope that this book will make even the most ardent bonded-composite enthusiast pause and think. The glass-ionomer cements are dynamic materials capable of renewing their bonds to dentine in the event of failure of isolated bonds. Their ability to ion-exchange at the tooth interface and to leach fluoride makes them the materials of choice for controlling dental caries in dentine. Composite materials after polymerization are inert and cannot renew any broken dentine bonds. Their great advantage lies in their enamel bonding using the acid-etch technique and this is where they should be used, as enamel replacements.

This atlas highlights the importance of having a basic understanding of the science of materials if the practitioner is to use them to maximum advantage. I am certain that students and dentists will enjoy looking over Graham Mount's shoulder as he reveals his successes and failures in clinical practice over many years with these challenging polyelectrolyte cements.

John W McLean, OBE
FDS, MDS, DSc, D ODONT, Clinical Consultant,
Laboratory of The Government Chemist,
London

Preface

An article by Alan Wilson in the *British Dental Journal* in 1972 concerning a new cement for dentistry stirred further thoughts on developing dental materials. The requirements of an ideal restorative material are not difficult to define and have been itemized often. Any material which begins to approach this ideal should be further investigated, and I waited with interest for the next stage.

Its formal introduction to the market was undertaken by John McLean at an Australian Dental Congress held in Adelaide 4 years later, after he had conducted an intensive period of clinical testing. The usual brief period of euphoria followed and no one dared leave the Congress without their box of ASPA. However, the profession has a bad habit of equating new materials with old and expects them to behave in the same way. If it does not pack like amalgam and look like composite resin, then it is a problem. In this case the old adage, 'when all else fails read the instructions' was of little benefit because the instructions were very poorly written. The result for the average practitioner was a disaster, and nothing switches a practitioner off quite so quickly as two failures in a row. He or she will accept the blame for one, but the second time it fails, it has to be the material at fault and not the practitioner.

Simple laboratory investigations showed where the main problems lay, but the negative outlook engendered by the early experiences was hard to overcome. Fortunately, a number of manufacturers took an interest and worked on upgrading the material. Over a period of time the glass-ionomer system has become quite sophisticated and a very valuable addition to our armamentarium. More manufacturers are now entering the field, but they must be aware that the chemistry of these materials is rather sophisticated and not easily copied. The principle advantages that cannot be lost or overlooked are: the ionic exchange with tooth structure available through the poly(alkenoic acid), and the fluoride release for remineralization. Some of the newer cements appear to be drifting from the original formula and, therefore, will not belong in this group of cements.

There is still room for improvement and, hopefully, the chemists in dental materials research will be able to increase the fracture strength of these materials and stabilize them against water exchange during early setting procedures. In addition, further clinical research is required to develop straightforward guidelines for the practitioner to ensure success with placement.

This handbook is designed to offer the clinician the current status of clinical placement. The routines described herein have been developed over the last 12 years and continuing observation would suggest that longevity in the oral environment is not a problem, provided always that the material is not subjected to undue occlusal load.

For a deeper study of the basic science of the glass-ionomer cements, the reader is referred to the textbook by Wilson and McLean. This is the definitive treatise on the subject and will be frequently quoted in this text as the original authority. The present book is devoted entirely to the clinical aspects and is meant to be utilized as an instant guide in the clinical situation. Special chapters are set aside for dental assistants, on the premise that they need to know at least as much as their operator to ensure that patients get full measure out of all known dental materials.

GJM

Acknowledgments

My initial interest was stimulated by an article written by Alan Wilson in the *British Dental Journal* of 1972, followed by meeting both Alan Wilson and John McLean in London. I was then most fortunate in my own dental school to have Dr Owen Makinson, who encouraged me and made it possible for me to continue clinical research in the materials laboratory. His talent for lateral thinking can be both confusing and enlightening but the end result is almost always clarification. The ability to examine in the laboratory what I was attempting at the chairside, and vice versa, was both stimulating and encouraging. This was combined with continuing contact with John McLean who explained, at a scientific level, observations I had made clinically but lacked the knowledge to understand.

Two other giants in the dental materials world, Ralph Phillips and Dennis Smith, have been most tolerant and understanding of my lack of scientific background and have supported my work very generously. Exchange of information between disciplines is, of course, essential and we are very fortunate to have scientists of their stature devoting their interests to the assessment and development of dental materials.

The manufacturers of dental materials also have a responsibility to the profession and our patients. They do much of the developmental research these days and the profession, in fact, carries out many of their field studies. It is imperative, therefore, that we keep in touch, and I must acknowledge my appreciation and gratitude to GC International, Japan, and ESPE, Germany, for their continued support and interest. I have always tried to avoid being identified with any particular product or company because it is very easy for a bias to show and I think then a researcher may run the risk of losing validity. However, these two companies have, in my opinion, devoted more time to the development of the glass-ionomer cements than any other, and their products show it.

There are many others, of course, who have supported and assisted me in my professional career. I shall always be grateful to Dr Gilbert Brinsden, former Chairman of Fixed Prosthodontics, Northwestern University Dental School, Chicago, who, in effect, 'opened the door' to international dentistry for me. I must acknowledge my patients, who have been very tolerant of having their restorations photographed, and my staff, who have learned new techniques, appeared in my videos and kept my records. I have also been fortunate in being able to utilize the services of two very able laboratory technicians, John Friemanis and Norman Lee, whose expertise and good humour have been invaluable over all these years. I would also like to thank the following for photographic work: Dr GS Heithersay (Figures 3.45–3.49) Dr W Kullman (Figures 5.10–5.14 and 6.37–6.40) and Dr R Smales (Figure 1.7 and 1.8). Many members of the Faculty of Dentistry of the University of Adelaide have assisted in many ways, and South Australian Dental Services have been very generous in allowing me access to the dental building and all its facilities.

However, none of this would have been possible without the support of my family, in particular, my wife. We have shared a study for many years, one at the sewing machine and the other on the dictation machine. I am grateful indeed for her tolerance. She is now a very good seamstress.

Sources

Some illustrations have already been published and are reproduced here with kind permission:

Clarke JW, ed, *Clinical Dentistry* (Harper and Row: New York 1984) vol 4, chap 20A: Figures 1.9, 1.10;

Mount GJ, Glass-ionomer cements: obtaining optimum aesthetic results, *Dental Outlook* (1988) **14** iii: 3–6: Figures 1.9, 1.10, 1.13, 1.14, 1.17;

Mount GJ, Clinical requirements for a successful 'sandwich' – dentine to glass-ionomer cement to composite resin, *Aust Dent J* (in press): Figures 1.16, 5.3–5.6, 5.17, 5.19, 5.21;

Mount GJ, Glass-ionomer cements in gerodontics. A status report for the American Journal of Dentistry, *Am J Dent* (1988) **1**: 123–8: Figures 6.47–6.52.

1 Description of glass-ionomer cements

The glass-ionomer cements are water-based cements, probably more accurately known as glass-polyalkenoate cements. They consist of an alumino-silicate glass with a high fluoride content, interacted with a poly(alkenoic acid). The result is a cement consisting of glass particles surrounded and supported by a matrix arising from the dissolution of the surface of the glass particles in the acid. Calcium polyacrylate chains form quite rapidly following mixing of the two components, and develop the initial matrix which holds the particles together. Once the calcium ions are involved, the aluminium ions will begin to form aluminium polyacrylate chains and, as these are less soluble and notably stronger, the final matrix formation takes place. This matrix is relatively insoluble in oral fluids but, as the fluoride droplets present are not part of the matrix system, the ability to release fluoride ions into the surrounding tooth structure and saliva is retained.

The fluoride is used initially as a flux in the manufacture of the glass particles and has been shown to be an essential part of the setting reaction. It represents approximately 20 per cent of the final glass in the form of minute droplets. These become available from the matrix more readily than they were from the original glass particles.

Approximately 24 per cent of the set cement is water and, at least until the formation of the aluminium polyacrylate chains is well advanced, further water can be taken up by the water-soluble calcium polyacrylate chains. Alternatively, if the cement is allowed to remain exposed to air, then water will be lost. This problem of water loss or water uptake, that is, water balance, is probably the most important and least understood problem with this group of cements (Figures 1.1, 1.2).

From the clinical point of view, it is this property alone which dictates the handling characteristics of each of the classifications of these cements. The chemical reaction initiated by the application of poly(alkenoic acid) to the surface of the glass particles is, in fact, very prolonged. The initial set will reach a stage within 4 minutes at which it is possible to remove a matrix and carry out trimming of the newly-placed restoration. However, complete maturity and resistance to water loss will not be available for at least 2 weeks for the fast-setting varieties and possibly 6 months for the slow-setting aesthetic cements.

If it is necessary to allow the cement to come into contact with water within minutes of placement, then a fast-set cement is required. However, achievement of rapid resistance to water uptake can only be gained with the sacrifice of aesthetics. In the manufacturing process, excess calcium ions are stripped from the surface of the glass particles so that the aluminium ion exchange will commence earlier in the life of the cement. Ultimate physical properties will not be reduced but translucency is lost.

However, it must be recognized that this early resistance to water uptake does not lock the water in, and all of the fast-setting cements remain subject to dehydration. This means that, when using them as a lining, for example, they should not be left exposed to air any longer than is necessary, since the cement is likely to crack.

If it is important to achieve an aesthetic end result in the restoration, then acceleration of the setting procedure is not possible and the clinician must accept the resultant problems of maintaining a stable environment for the newly-placed restoration. Considerable water uptake and water loss can occur in these cements for at least 1 hour and may continue for a further 24 hours on a reducing scale. Thereafter, water uptake is of less significance although water loss will remain a problem. If a relatively young restoration is to be exposed

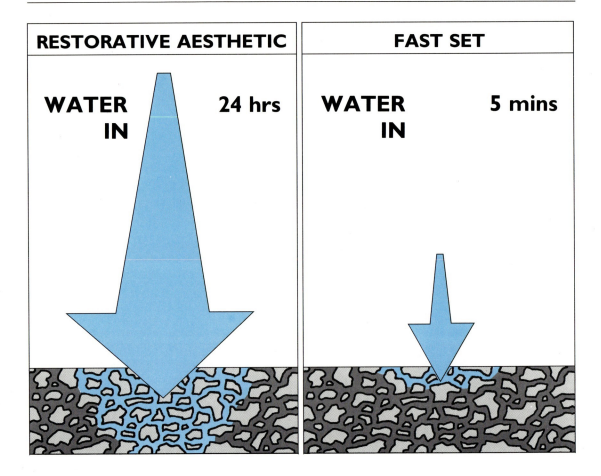

Figure 1.1

Diagrammatic representation of the water balance in the glass-ionomer cements. Restorative aesthetic cements remain susceptible to water uptake for at least 1 day after placement. Fast-setting cements are resistant to water uptake within 5 minutes of the beginning of mix.

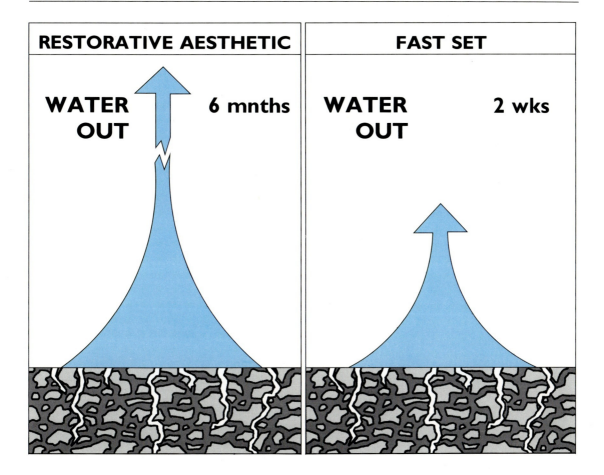

Figure 1.2

The problem of water loss continues for a longer period for both the fast- and the slow-set varieties and precautions must be taken to prevent dehydration.

again to dehydration in the first 6 months after placement, it should be sealed with a waterproof coating to minimize water exchange.

Considerable effort is being expended at present on overcoming these problems of water balance. It has been suggested that the profession is intolerant of the time taken up by the setting reaction and that faster-setting cements, particularly lining cements, are necessary. Certainly conservation of time is important during clinical placement, but it is even more imperative that the inherent advantages of chemical union to enamel and dentine, as well as that of continuing fluoride release, are not reduced or eliminated in the process.

The term 'glass-ionomer cement' should not be loosely applied to a material simply because it contains an ionomer glass. Now on the market, there are materials for cavity lining which are light activated, enabling placement in the cavity and setting within 20–30 seconds using the usual light wand. Other restorative materials can then be placed over them immediately. Providing they consist basically of a high fluoride ionomer glass with a poly(alkenoic acid), then it is possible that the development of the polyacrylate chains will still occur and chelation with tooth structure and fluoride release will therefore be available. However, the clinical application of the present first generation light-activated glass-ionomer cements should be restricted to lining a cavity followed by complete coverage with another restorative material (see Chapter 5). Fluoride release will then be restricted to the dentine of the restored tooth only. They contain up to 10 per cent resin to allow for the initial light-activated setting reaction and at present the extent to which this may alter or modify the development of the polyacrylic chains is unknown.

The initial setting reaction, developed under the influence of the light, leads to a firm consistency but it takes up to 24 hours before they are set hard and have developed their full physical properties. Care should be exercised in submitting them to stress during this period. Further clinical and laboratory research is needed to define properly their place in clinical practice, but there is no doubt that providing they are not exposed to the oral environment they represent a safe, rapidly placed lining material (see page 67).

Other available materials contain an ionomer glass with no poly(alkenoic acid), or with additional ingredients which tend to alter the chemistry. These do not fit into the category of glass-ionomer cements and are not discussed further here.

Classification

The following classification is adapted from Wilson and McLean (1988). It is generally accepted and will be used throughout this book.

Type I Luting cements
- For cementation of crowns, bridges and inlays.
- Powder/liquid ratio approximately 1.5:1.
- Fast set with early resistance to water uptake.
- Ultimate film thickness 25 μ or less.
- Radiopaque.

Type II Restorative
II.1 Restorative aesthetic
- For any application requiring an aesthetic restoration; the only limitation is no undue occlusal load.
- Powder/liquid ratio, 2.5:1 to 6.8:1.
- Good shade range.
- Prolonged setting reaction and therefore remains subject to water uptake and water loss for at least 24 hours after placement; requires immediate protection from the oral environment.
- Radiolucent (most brands).

II.2 Restorative reinforced
- For use where aesthetic considerations are not important but rapid set and high physical properties are required.
- Powder/liquid ratio 3:1 to 4:1.
- Rapid set with early resistance to water uptake and can therefore be polished immediately after placement; remains susceptible to dehydration for 2 weeks after initial set.
- Radiopaque.

Type III Lining cements
- For use as a standard lining material under all other restorative materials and is particularly recommended to provide dentine adhesion for composite resin.
- Powder/liquid ratio 1.5:1 to 4:1.
- Physical properties increase as powder content increases.
- Lacks aesthetic properties.
- Radiopaque.

Significant factors

Powder/liquid ratio

It is important to be aware that the constituents of the various glass-ionomer cements on the market are not the same. There is, in fact, a considerable difference between the powders and liquids produced by various manufacturers, and products must therefore never be interchanged. It should also be noted that, in some cases, materials marketed under different names are made by the same manufacturer.

The heat history of the glass during manufacture has a bearing on the clinical handling and ultimate physical properties of the cement. The glass powders, in the earlier formulations in particular, are of a high fluoride variety to allow for a rapid setting reaction, and these glasses are rather opaque. Another method of speeding the setting reaction is to deplete the available calcium ions on the surface of the powder. This also will be at the expense of aesthetics, but will result in a cement with an early resistance to water uptake. The introduction of tartaric acid into the formula to speed up the setting reaction led to the use of glasses of lower fluoride content, which are notably more translucent, and these are particularly valuable in the Type II.I restorative aesthetic cements.

Powder particle size varies between both manufacturers and cement types. Generally, the slower-setting aesthetic cements have particles ranging up to 50 μ in size, while the faster-setting luting and lining cements have a finer particle distribution. Smaller particle size speeds the chemical reaction, and also improves the chance of achieving a fine film thickness.

In the original formula, the liquid was a poly-(acrylic acid) and this posed difficulties. Higher molecular weight and concentration of acid increases strength and accelerates setting time. However, the viscosity of the liquid also increases as the molecular weight goes up and clinical handling becomes difficult. In addition, the viscosity of the acid tends to increase during storage, which makes dispensing and mixing more difficult still. Subsequently, copolymers of acrylic acid with other unsaturated carboxylic acids, such as itaconic acid and maleic acid, were developed, and these proved more reliable, easily handled and stored. As long as the polyacid is present in solution, however, the problem of increased viscosity with an increase in molecular weight or concentration remains. Hence the present trend towards utilizing a dehydrated form of polyacid and incorporating it in the powder, using either water or dilute tartaric acid as the liquid. The resultant mixed cement has a relatively low viscosity and is therefore easier to handle and is particularly suitable as a luting cement.

Because, in the anhydrous form, acids of a higher molecular weight can be incorporated, the physical properties of these cements are generally superior. Certainly, shelf life is improved, hand-mixing on a glass slab is easier and a fine film thickness can be achieved more readily with the luting cements.

As with all dental restorative materials, the powder/liquid ratio has a significant bearing on ultimate physical properties. To a certain extent, the greater the amount of powder the higher the ultimate properties. However, where there is insufficient liquid to wet the powder particles, a point will be reached where translucency will decline, in the presence of unreacted particles.

Lower powder ratios are required with the luting cements so that optimum film thickness can be achieved. Also, when using the cement in small quantities as a lining under other restorative materials, such as amalgam or gold, it is more readily handled with a lower powder content, and physical properties will not be of great significance. However, if it is to be a base under composite resin, then physical properties will be significant and a high powder/liquid ratio is indicated.

Hand-mixing of these cements is possible, but considerable variation in the powder content will result unless extreme care is taken in measuring out when dispensing. Hand-mixing at the higher powder/liquid ratios for the restorative cements is very difficult, and capsulation is strongly recommended as being the ideal method of dispensing. The powder/liquid ratio can be standardized, as well as the mixing time and, therefore, the setting time. Ultimate physical properties will then not be in doubt.

When mixing mechanically, care must be taken to see that the correct time is used according to the machine available. Manufacturers generally suggest 10 seconds with a machine capable of 4000 cycles/min. These are generally known as 'ultra-high-speed' amalgamators, but some machines will produce up to nearly 5000 cycles/min and may therefore over-mix and reduce working time.

The estimation of effective working time can be made by determining the 'loss of gloss' of the newly

BOX A   MIXING OF CAPSULES

Trituration of capsules of glass-ionomer cements is not necessarily a straightforward procedure. Manufacturers give a recommended time for capsules in a so-called high-energy amalgamator, but it must be realized that not all amalgamators are the same and, probably more important still, all amalgamators can vary in the amount of energy dispensed on any given day.

A high-speed amalgamator works at approximately 3000 cycles/min.

Ultra-high-speed amalgamators work at approximately 4500 cycles/min.

However, the number of cycles may vary by as much as 10 per cent on either side of this figure under normal circumstances, and factors such as ambient temperature, power surges, manufacturer variation, and age of the machine can produce much greater differences. The operator should therefore be prepared to check the state of the mix periodically to ensure a predictable and standard result.

Check the efficiency of your machine by assessing the 'loss of gloss' of a freshly mixed capsule.

Determining the 'loss of gloss'

- Mix a capsule for 10 seconds and express the contents onto a glass slab in a single pile. Start the timer (*a*).

- The material will have a wet glossy surface and will slump down on the slab without spreading out.
- Using a dental probe or small instrument, touch the top of the pile and lift the cement up. It should string up 2.0 cm or so from the top, then break away and slump back to its original shape (*b,c*).
- At some point, the glossy surface will begin to dull. The material will no longer string out as far as before, nor will it slump to its original form (*d*).
- Note the time. Subtract 15 seconds, and the remainder is the effective working time available at that mixing time with that machine.
- Vary the mixing time as required to set the correct working time for your situation.
- Extending the mixing time may produce a mix that will flow better, but the rise in temperature produced by the increase in energy expended may reduce the working time quite dramatically.
- Reducing the mixing time may produce a mix that will flow more readily because not all the liquid has been utilized. Working and setting time will then be considerably extended but physical properties will be downgraded.

Bass EV, Wing G, The mixing of encapsulated glass-ionomer cement restorative materials, *Aust Dent J* (1988) **33**:243.

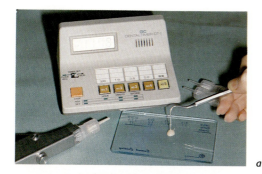
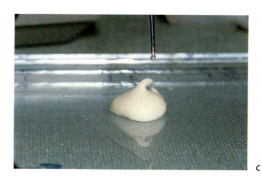
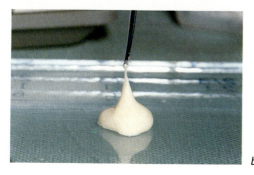
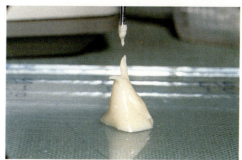

Determining the 'loss of gloss' (see Box A).

mixed material (see Box A, page 6). Careful observation of a sample mix will show when the gloss goes off, and placement of the cement after that point will risk failure. Working time should be at least 2 minutes from the completion of mix and this will normally be achieved with a mixing time of 7–10 seconds. A shorter mixing time may leave unreacted liquid visible in the cement, while a longer period will result in an unacceptably short working time.

There is a degree of porosity incorporated in all of these cements which is unavoidable. There appears to be a greater variation in the size of porosities when the cement is hand mixed. Machine-mixed capsulated cement demonstrates similar porosity but the voids are uniformly smaller. Surface porosity will result, on occasion, in uptake of surface stain.

Time to mature

The setting reaction of the glass-ionomer cements can be described as an ionic cross-linking between polyacid chains, giving a rigidly bound polyacid/salt matrix. The initial cross-linking involves the more readily available calcium ions, producing an early set to allow removal of the matrix. However, these divalent linkages are not stable and are readily soluble in water. The setting reaction continues within the hard cement mass with further cross-linking by the less-soluble trivalent aluminium ions. This second phase produces an increase in physical properties, along with a reduction in solubility, resulting in a hard, stable, brittle material with a highly-linked polyacid/salt matrix. It is possible to increase the speed of this reaction, with a dramatic reduction in the time taken for the development

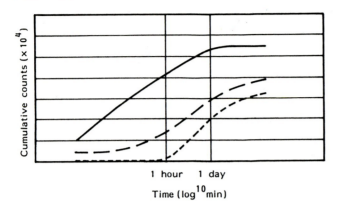

Figure 1.3

Relative efficiency of proprietary varnishes and single-component, low-viscosity, light-activated bonding resin as sealants, maintaining water balance within the cement. The resin bond gives more water retention at 24 hours and therefore better physical properties and greater translucency.

——————— Control
— — — Proprietary varnish
- - - Low-viscosity, light-cured resin bonding agent

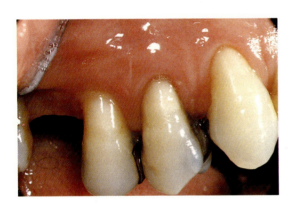

Figure 1.4

Class V glass-ionomer cement restorations in the upper-right canine and both bicuspids, 5 years after placement. They were sealed with a very low viscosity, light-activated bonding resin and display excellent colour and translucency.

of the calcium polyacrylate chains and therefore an early resistance to water uptake and lowered solubility.

The rapid setting time can only be achieved at the expense of colour and translucency so that, if a Type II.1 restorative aesthetic cement is to be utilized, to obtain optimum results it is necessary to protect the setting cement against water uptake for some hours after placement. In certain materials, physical properties at 15 minutes may be sufficient to be able to contour and polish the newly placed restorations. However, if disturbed at this point, there will be sufficient water uptake to reduce the translucency to unacceptable levels, as well as to lower the physical properties and the attachment to dentine.

The maintenance of water balance for 24 hours allows optimum development of aesthetics and is recommended (Figures 1.3, 1.4).

Manufacturers provide a varnish to seal the newly placed restoration from the oral environment, but this has proved to be less than ideal. The varnish has an evaporative vehicle incorporated in it and therefore porosities are likely to appear as the vehicle evaporates (Figure 1.5). If the varnish is carefully applied and the vehicle evaporated, followed by a second coat carefully blown dry, a reasonable result can be achieved. Careful drying should be carried out for approximately 30 seconds for each coat of varnish before allowing the restoration to get wet.

The most efficient seal can be obtained by using one of the single-component, very low-viscosity, light-activated, unfilled bonding resins, which are part of the composite resin system, instead of the varnish (Figure 1.6). It has been shown that lower

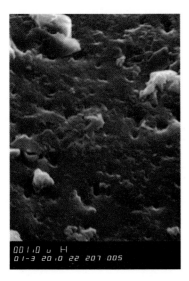

Figure 1.5

SEM of proprietary varnish recommended for sealing glass-ionomer cements. Note the relative porosity. *Original magnification* x 1000.

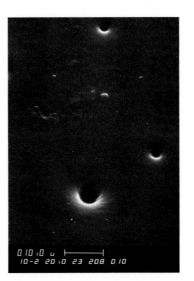

Figure 1.6

SEM of single-component very low viscosity, light-activated resin bonding agent. Note the lack of porosity. *Original magnification* x 1000.

viscosity permits better adaptation of the resin to the cement surface, and therefore a better seal. Bonding agents which need to be premixed and contain an evaporative vehicle to reduce their viscosity will not be effective because they are likely to be porous when set, therefore allowing water exchange through the resin film. The same applies to chemically activated bonding agents which, of course, require hand-mixing, with the consequent potential for incorporation of air bubbles and porosities (Figures 1.7–1.16).

Recent work has shown that the layer of bonding resin will remain on the surface of the restoration for some time, depending upon the vigour of the patient's brushing routine. Using a specially-prepared Visio-Bond containing a fluorescent dye, specimens have been monitored for as long as 6 weeks and have shown a reasonable quantity of resin still in place on the cement. In view of the prolonged chemical maturation

which occurs with glass-ionomer cements, the continued presence of the resin is desirable.

It should be noted that, if a new restoration less than 6 months old is to be exposed to dehydration for longer than a few minutes, it is desirable to protect it again with a further layer of unfilled resin bond. After 6 months, the cement is generally mature enough to withstand such stress (Figure 1.17).

The only problem arising from the use of such a long-lasting sealant is that, with a Class V restoration, an artificial overhang may be created and, with a Class III restoration, the contact area may be closed by the resin. Both situations should be anticipated and appropriate precautions taken. An overhang can be removed at the time of placement by using a sharp blade to cut away from the restoration towards the tooth (Figure 1.18). A closed contact can be re-opened later at the polishing appointment, if the patient has been

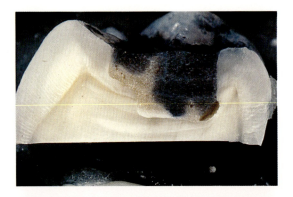

Figure 1.7

Class I glass-ionomer cement restoration, placed in the occlusal surface of an extracted molar tooth. It was covered with a proprietary varnish and immersed in dye 7 minutes after placement. There is severe penetration of the dye into the cement.

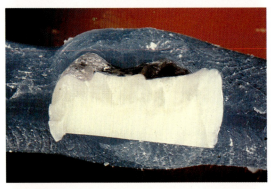

Figure 1.8

Similar restoration which has been sealed with a single-component low-viscosity, light-activated resin bonding agent. Note the complete lack of dye penetration.

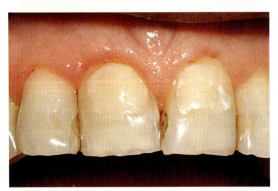

Figure 1.9

Glass-ionomer cement restorations on the labial surface of both upper-central incisors. The restoration on the left-central was placed 2 years prior to the right-central and was protected with a proprietary varnish. Note the white defect on the left-central.

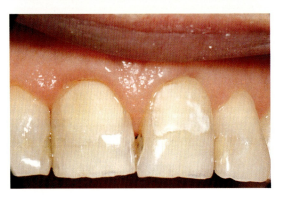

Figure 1.10

When the restorations are dried off, the white defect is more pronounced. However, the restoration in the right-central, which was protected at insertion with a light-activated resin bond, remains unaffected by dehydration.

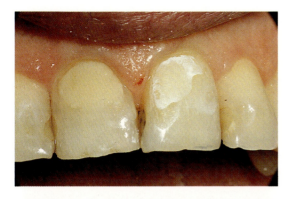

Figure 1.11

Polishing back the restoration in the left-central shows that the defect penetrates through the entire depth of the cement.

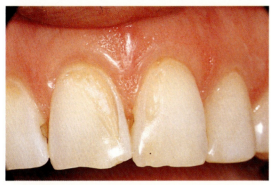

Figure 1.12

Labial erosion lesions on the two upper-central incisors before treatment.

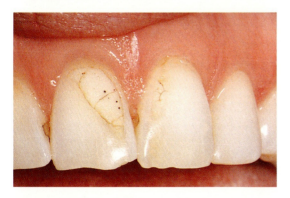

Figure 1.13

The lesions were restored with glass-ionomer cements 5 years prior to this photograph, and were protected at insertion with copal varnish only. They appear to have been both hydrated and dehydrated before maturing and require replacement.

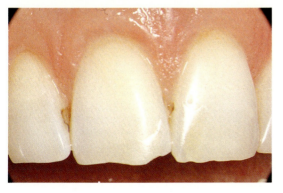

Figure 1.14

The restorations were replaced with another glass-ionomer cement and protected with a very low viscosity, light-activated bonding resin. They had been in place for 2 years when photographed.

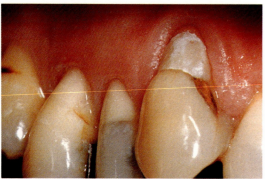

Figure 1.15

Three Class V restorations placed on different occasions. The restoration in the upper-right canine was placed 10 years ago and was not properly protected. It therefore remains subject to dehydration and lacks translucency. The two bicuspids were restored approximately 5 years ago and were properly protected.

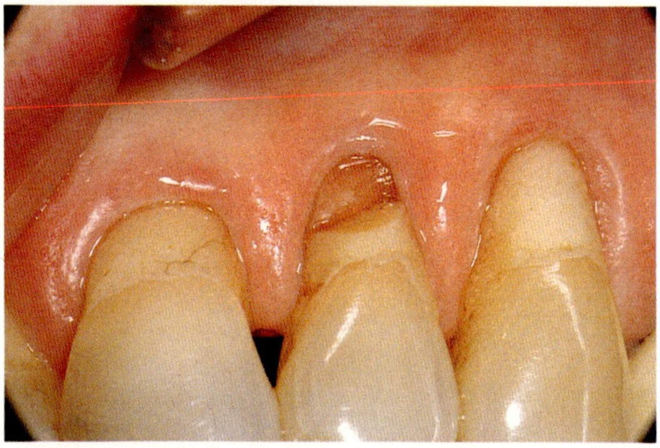

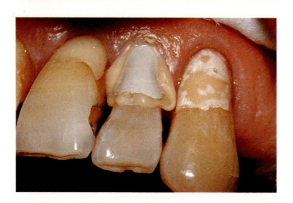

Figure 1.16

Class V restorations in the upper-left central and lateral incisors, both of which were allowed to dehydrate shortly after placement. The restoration in the central incisor is cracked and the one in the lateral has suffered bulk failure as a result.

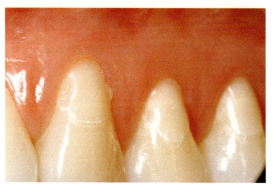

Figure 1.17

Class V restorations in the upper-left central, lateral and canine. The upper-central restoration has been in place for over 1 year and was properly protected. The restoration in the canine was placed 6 months previously and was regarded as mature. However, as the restoration was being placed in the lateral incisor, the cement in the canine dehydrated on the surface after approximately 10 minutes' exposure to air, showing that even at 6 months it was not completely mature.

Figure 1.18

Class V restorations were placed in the upper-left canine and both bicuspids 24 hours previously and they were protected with a generous coat of bonding resin. There are still small projections of resin remaining at the gingival margins, which may retain plaque and should be removed.

unable to remove the resin. Mostly, the patient will succeed in restoring freedom.

Most manufacturers maintain that their aesthetic restorative glass-ionomer cement can be contoured and polished at approximately 10–15 minutes after placement. Certainly, the cement will have achieved a degree of set such that polishing can be carried out, but only at the sacrifice of translucency and aesthetics. **Both water uptake and water loss within the first 24 hours will downgrade the physical properties and appearance** of all these cements, and it is well worth while delaying the final finish for at least a day – preferably a week – if optimum results are required (Figures 1.19–1.22).

It has been suggested in the past that it is necessary to cut a shallow finish line along the incisal margin of a Class V erosion lesion because the cement is likely to 'ditch' along that margin if left in thin section. However, providing the cement is protected as suggested with a completely waterproof sealant and is thus allowed to mature completely, then the cement will survive satisfactorily even though in thin section (Figure 1.21).

The chemistry of the fast-setting Type I, Type II reinforced and Type III cements has been modified to the extent that they are relatively resistant to water uptake within 5 minutes of the start of mix. They are, however, still subject to dehydration for up to 2 weeks after placement. If left exposed for 10 minutes, they will visibly crack and craze, and attachment to enamel and dentine will fail (Figure 1.23). If, for example, a quadrant of cavities has been exposed under rubber dam and glass-ionomer cement is to be used as a lining, the teeth should be restored one at a time. The lining is placed and, as soon as it is set, covered with the final restoration. If a Type II reinforced cement (for example, Ketac Silver) is to be used as the restoration, then it should be protected against dehydration with an unfilled resin bond while the remaining restorations are being placed. Once the cement is covered or is immersed in saliva, it is safe from further dehydration (Figure 1.24).

The corollary to this rapid-setting mechanism is that the Type II reinforced restoration (Ketac Silver) can be completed all the way to a final polish, beginning 6 minutes after the start of mix. Once the initial set is achieved, it can be contoured and polished to a very fine surface, using ultra-fine diamonds followed by graded rubber polishing points under air/water spray, taking care not to dehydrate.

Adhesion to enamel and dentine

Chemical bonding can be obtained between the cement and the dentine or enamel. Wilson has described an ionic-exchange layer which is visible under the scanning electron microscope and represents the chemical union between the two. Because of the relatively low tensile strength of the cement, failure of the union will normally occur within the cement rather than at the interface between the cement and the tooth (Figures 1.25, 1.26). This presupposes, however, that the interface is clear of debris such as saliva, pellicle, plaque, blood and other contaminants (Figures 1.27–1.29). In the clinical situation, this can be achieved by conditioning the cavity surface with a brief application of 10 per cent poly(acrylic acid). This is a relatively mild acid which will dissolve the smear layer within 15 seconds, although if left for longer than 20 seconds, it is likely to begin to demineralize remaining dentine and enamel and open up dentinal tubules. There are two additional advantages in using this particular material for conditioning the dentine. Firstly, as it is the acid utilized in the cement itself, any residue inadvertently left behind will not interfere in the setting reaction and, secondly, it has been suggested that the poly(acrylic acid) will pre-activate the calcium ions in the dentine and render them more available for ionic exchange with the cement (Wilson and McLean, 1988).

If chemical union is to be relied upon to retain the restoration in a Class V erosion cavity, it is recommended that the surface of the tooth be cleaned first with a slurry of pumice and water (Figures 1.30–1.32). Note that most proprietary polishing pastes will leave a smear layer behind, so plain pumice and water is preferred. The surface should now be conditioned with 10 per cent poly(acrylic acid) for 15 seconds. This will remove any remaining debris and pre-activate the calcium ions in the dentine (Figures 1.33, 1.34). No cavity preparation is required. On the other hand, if chemical adhesion is not required, as with a lining under amalgam or gold, then conditioning the dentine is an unnecessary step (Figure 1.35).

It should be noted that an alternative to removing the smear layer is to apply a mineralizing solution, such as Causton's ITS solution (see Box B) or 25 per cent tannic acid, which will tend to unite the smear layer to the underlying dentine and enamel and seal over dentinal tubules. This is the recommended technique when using glass-ionomer

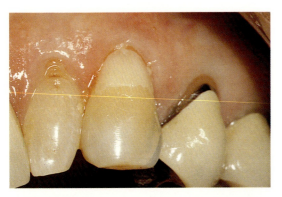

Figure 1.19

Class V restoration on the upper-left canine immediately after placement. Note the relative lack of translucency.

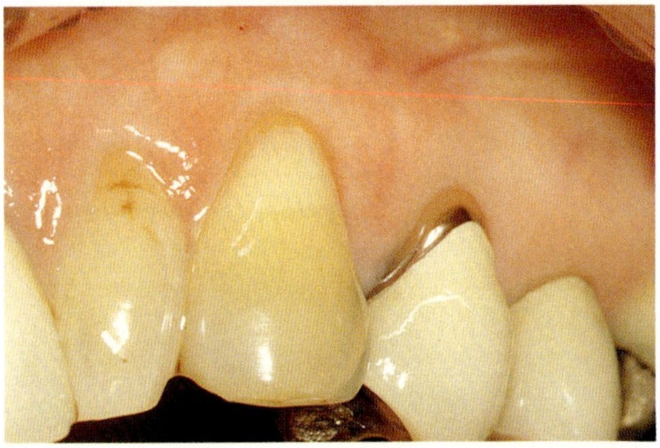

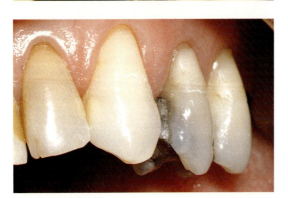

Figure 1.20

The same restoration following polishing, 1 week after placement. There is an improvement of colour match and translucency.

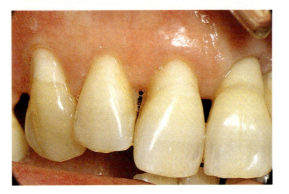

Figure 1.21

Class V erosion lesions in the upper left canine, first and second bicuspids were restored five years previously and protected with a resin-bonding agent. The restorations have not been polished at all and have retained the original surface from the matrix. Note also that even though a finish line was not cut in the dentine along the incisal margin, the excess 'flash' remains intact.

Figure 1.22

Class V glass-ionomer cement restorations in a group of upper anteriors, extending from the left-central incisor to the right canine, about 4 years after placement, showing complete maturity and stability.

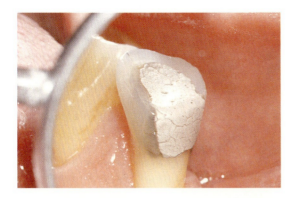

Figure 1.23

Class II Ketac Silver restoration which was not protected immediately after placement, while a further restoration was being placed in the second molar in the same quadrant. It was exposed to air for approximately 20 minutes and therefore dehydrated and cracked.

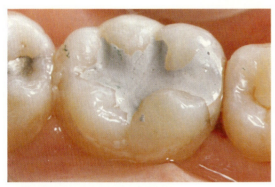

Figure 1.24

Class II Ketac Silver in a conventional cavity design about 3 years after placement. The patient does not exert a heavy occlusal load and the restoration is well maintained. It was polished before removal of the rubber dam and has maintained its surface finish well.

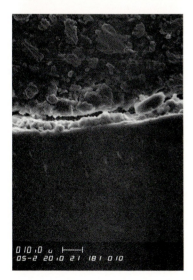

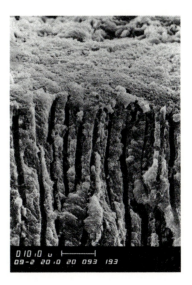

Figure 1.25

SEM showing the ionic-exchange layer between the glass-ionomer cement and the dentine. The layer is firmly adherent to the dentine and separation has occurred in the cement due to dehydration during preparation of the specimen for the SEM. *Original magnification* x 500.

Figure 1.26

SEM showing the ionic-exchange layer remaining on the dentine after complete loss of the cement. *Original magnification* x 900.

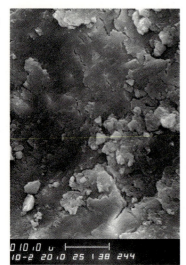

Figure 1.27

SEM showing the smear layer left on the dentine surface following cavity preparation at slow speed. Note that in the oral cavity there will be an admixture of plaque, pellicle, saliva and blood. If the ionic-exchange layer is to be developed (Figure 1.25), the smear layer should be removed. *Original magnification* x 1000.

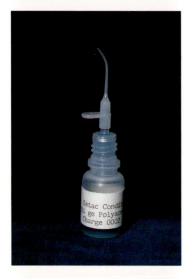

Figure 1.28

Dropper bottle used for the application of 10 per cent poly(acrylic acid). The lumen occasionally may be occluded by the acid setting in it, but can be washed out.

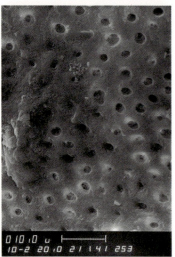

Figure 1.29

SEM showing the surface of the dentine after a 15-second application of 10 per cent poly(acrylic acid). Note that many of the dentine tubules are still occluded but the surface is relatively clean. *Original magnification* x 900.

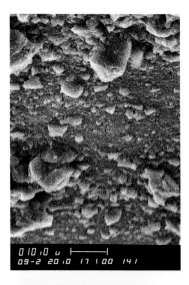

Figure 1.30

SEM showing the surface of an erosion lesion prior to cleaning. The accumulated plaque will inhibit the development of the required ion-exchange layer. *Original magnification* x 900.

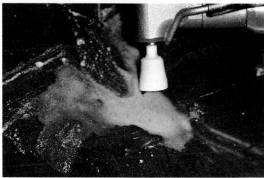

Figure 1.31

Slurry of pumice in water. This is the preferred material for removing plaque from the surface of an erosion lesion.

Figure 1.32

SEM of an erosion lesion after cleaning with a slurry of pumice in water for 5 seconds. Note that generally all the dentinal tubules are closed over by burnished dentine. *Original magnification* x 900.

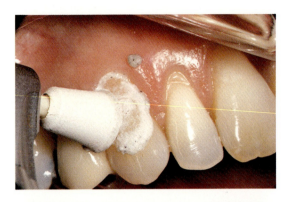

Figure 1.33

Cleaning an erosion lesion with a slurry of pumice in water.

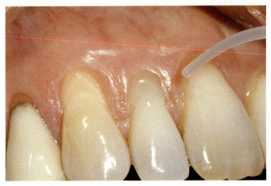

Figure 1.34

Conditioning the surface with 10 per cent poly(acrylic acid), following cleaning. The area should be washed thoroughly after 10–15 seconds.

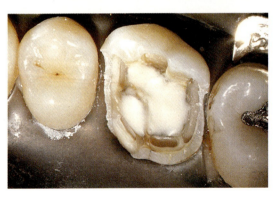

Figure 1.35

Glass-ionomer cement placed as a lining under an amalgam restoration. It is 0.5 mm thick and covers the pulpal floor only.

BOX B   CAUSTON'S ITS SOLUTION

The following is the formula for the mineralizing solution recommended for attaching the smear layer on to the dentine and sealing dentinal tubules. This solution can be made up by a pharmacist and is chemically stable for 18 months and longer.

Component	g/litre
$CaCl_2$	0.20
KCl	0.20
$MgCl.6H_2O$	0.05
NaCl	8.00
$NaHCO_3$	1.00
$NaH_2PO_4.H_2O$	0.05
Glucose	1.00

Adapted from Causton BE, Johnson NW, Improvement of polycarboxylate adhesion to dentine by the use of a new calcifying solution, *Br Dent J* (1982) **152**:9–11.

cement as a luting agent for full crowns. Considerable hydraulic pressure may be generated during the seating of crowns, and it is better to seal the tubules rather than open them up prior to placement. A 2-minute application of either Causton's ITS solution or 25 per cent tannic acid will offer protection and help to prevent post-insertion sensitivity.

Fluoride release

As with silicate cement, fluoride is used as a flux during the manufacture of the glass powder and it is then incorporated within the glass in the form of extremely fine droplets. Some fluoride is available from the powder particles themselves, but there is a considerable release following mixing with poly(alkenoic acid), and a continuing flow out of the matrix is available for long periods of time after placement. As the fluoride is not a part of the matrix of the cement, the fluoride release is not deleterious to the physical properties. It has been suggested that there is, in fact, a fluoride exchange available, with fluoride ions returning to the cement from external applications of fluoride at a later date if the fluoride gradient is in the right direction. Thus topical fluoride and the use of a fluoride toothpaste may provide a 'topping-up' effect.

In the presence of continuing fluoride release, plaque is less likely to accumulate on the surface of the restoration and, as there is no microleakage at the margin, both tissue tolerance and colour stability are of a very high order (Figure 1.36).

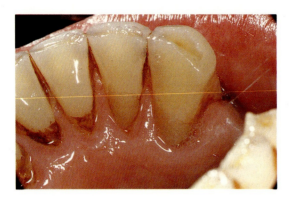

Figure 1.36

Class V glass-ionomer cement restorations on the lingual of the lower-left lateral and canine. There is an accumulation of calculus and plaque on the adjacent teeth and a relative lack of accumulation on the cement.

Pulp compatibility

The reasons for the high level of pulp compatibility are not entirely clear. However, it is suggested that the large size of the long-chain molecule reduces the ability of the acid to penetrate dentinal tubules (Wilson and McLean, 1988). In addition, dentine itself is a very effective buffer to acid attack. If there is 0.5 mm or more of remaining dentine over the pulp, then there would appear to be no pulpal irritation resulting from the presence of glass-ionomer cement. If there is any possibility of direct access to the pulp, then a small quantity of fast-setting calcium hydroxide can be placed in the immediate area where an exposure is suspected. The area to be covered should be kept to a minimum so as not to interfere with the chemical union between the cement and the dentine (Figure 1.37).

Physical properties

Work is in progress on increasing the physical properties of the glass-ionomer cements and it is anticipated that the next generation will extend the clinical applications of this group of materials quite markedly. Theoretically, flexural strength can be improved by the inclusion of a disperse phase, and this has been tried but is not yet clinically proven. Amalgam alloy particles have been added

but, as there is no union between the metal and the cement, physical properties remain virtually unaltered. The inclusion of very finely powdered pure silver particles, which are sintered to the surface of the glass powder, has been shown to produce a notable improvement in abrasion resistance. However, other physical properties are only moderately improved and, in fact, adhesion to dentine and enamel may be slightly reduced.

Variations to the basic constituents of the glass-ionomer cements are being subjected to experimentation and increases in physical properties may result. However, the essential elements of this group of cements will always be the ionic bond available between the cement and tooth structure through the presence of poly(alkenoic acid), as well as the fluoride release. Inclusions in the formula which reduce the effectiveness of the poly(alkenoic acid) or, indeed, eliminate the acid entirely will remove that cement from this highly successful group of restorative materials. There have been some lining cements released on the market recently which consist of a high fluoride ionomer glass incorporated in a light-activated resin. These are not glass-ionomer cements (see page 4).

Fracture resistance

At the present stage of development, the physical strength of the material is sufficient to withstand

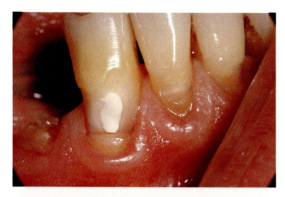

Figure 1.37

Very deep erosion on the lower-right canine which almost involved the pulp chamber. A limited area of fast-set calcium hydroxide has been laid down in the vicinity of the pulp chamber, leaving only the remainder of the dentine for ionic bonding with the cement.

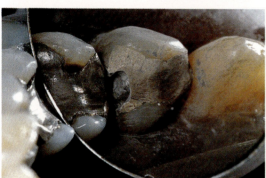

Figure 1.38

Large MOD Ketac Silver restoration in a lower-left first bicuspid. The occlusal load was heavier than anticipated and the distal marginal ridge has failed.

moderate occlusal load, provided it is well supported by surrounding tooth structure. It is not recommended for rebuilding cusps or marginal ridges to any extent, particularly in the patient who is likely to exert heavy occlusal stress (Figure 1.38). Resistance to tensile and shear stresses is such that it should not be relied upon as sole support for a crown, for example. The Type II.2 restorative reinforced version is valuable as a core build-up because it is possible to proceed immediately to the final preparation of the tooth. However, the cement requires considerable support itself from remaining tooth structure (Figure 1.39).

Resistance to shear stress is not good. For example, although it has an excellent record for the restoration of erosion lesions, it will not be retained on the labial surface of lower anterior teeth which have been abraded through a deep overbite and then suffered further erosion. Although there is room for the cement without interfering with the occlusion, the shear stresses are too great (Figure 1.40).

Abrasion resistance

The degradation of the material in the oral cavity has yet to be studied fully, but longevity studies suggest that a well-placed glass-ionomer cement will stand heavy abrasion better than remaining tooth structure, provided that the powder/liquid ratio is high enough (Mount, 1986) (Figure 1.41).

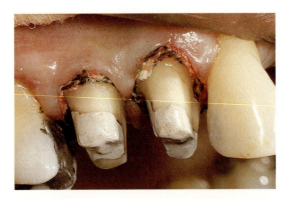

Figure 1.39

Core build-ups in Ketac Silver on two upper-right bicuspids. There is still sufficient natural tooth structure left to accept the occlusal load, thus compensating for the relative lack of tensile strength in the cement.

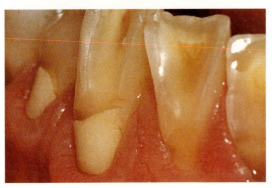

Figure 1.40

Three lower anteriors in a patient with a very deep overbite. Considerable abrasion has removed all the enamel and subsequently the dentine has been subjected to erosion. As there was sufficient space available, glass-ionomer cement restorations were placed on all three, but they all failed because of the extreme shear stresses. The only surviving cement is the gingival section on the canine, which was beyond the incisal edge of the opposing canine and therefore free of direct stress.

The presence of finely powdered silver particles on the surface of the glass, as in the Type II.2 restorative reinforced cement, will increase abrasion resistance to the stage where it is similar to amalgam and composite resin.

Radiopacity

It is possible to build radiopacity into the cements but only at the expense of aesthetics. Where the material is placed in such a position that further monitoring of its success must be carried out radiographically then, of course, it is essential that it be radiopaque. On the other hand, if it can be visually monitored and an aesthetic result is desirable, then radiopacity need not be incorporated (Figure 1.42).

Polishing

The process of producing a fine surface on any restorative material is one of reducing the depth of the scratches which have developed during recontouring. With the glass-ionomer cements, the smoothest surface will be that developed under the matrix. The surface will be mildly porous and matrix-rich, with very few glass particles showing and, prior to full maturity, very susceptible to damage. As far as possible, particularly early in the life of the restoration, any reshaping should be kept to a minimum and the surface developed by the matrix should be maintained. The cement can be trimmed lightly with a sharp blade, moving from the restoration toward the tooth. If the restoration is a Type II.1 restorative aesthetic cement, it should be sealed at this point and further polishing

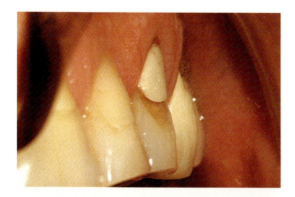

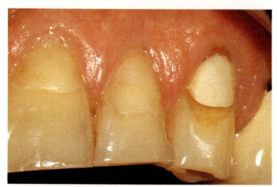

Figure 1.41

a Class V ASPA restoration in an upper-left canine, 12 years after placement. There is further erosion in the tooth structure beyond the cement restoration. Despite the rather poor quality cement, it has maintained its contour well.

b Same restoration as *a*. The restorations in the central and lateral incisors have been in place for 4 years.

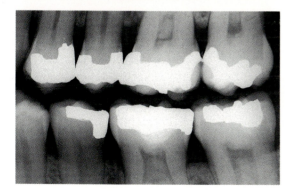

Figure 1.42

Tunnel restorations in the upper-right first and second molars showing that the radiopacity is very similar to amalgam.

delayed at least 24 hours. The other fast-setting cements can be contoured straight away. Any additional work that must be carried out with rotary instruments should be done under air/water spray to avoid dehydration of the cement.

Gross recontour can be achieved with a very fine diamond, and the surface refined with graded rubber abrasive polishing cups and points. A final finish will be gained with very fine, graded polishing disks (see Box C).

BOX C   POLISHING METHODS

Type II.1 restorative aesthetic
- Because of the slow-setting chemistry, do not attempt to contour or polish the cement for at least 24 hours.
- Gross contour can be achieved with very fine sintered diamonds under air/water spray at 20 000 revolutions/min.
- Refine the surface with graded rubber polishing points and cups at 5000 revolutions/min under air/water spray.
- Finish to a gloss with graded polishing discs at 3000 revolutions/min under air/water spray.

Type II.2 restorative reinforced
- Because of the rapid-setting chemistry, these cements can be contoured and polished beginning at 6 minutes from the start of mix.
- Gross contour can be achieved with very fine sintered diamonds under air/water spray at 20 000 revolutions/min.
- Refine the surface with graded rubber polishing points and cups at 5000 revolutions/min under air/water spray.

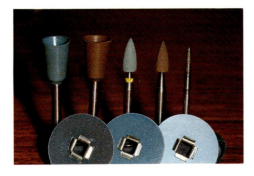

A selection of polishing cups and points, finishing and polishing discs.

2 Type I: Luting cements

Description

The chemistry of the luting cements is essentially the same as the others in this group of materials. However, the size of the powder particles is finer, to ensure achievement of an ultimate film thickness at an acceptable level. This involves compromise in that, with the finer particle size, working and setting times are reduced but physical properties are improved. Flow properties are such that placement of a restoration to its full extent is relatively easy and, unlike the zinc phosphate cements, it is unnecessary to maintain positive pressure on the restoration during the setting period (Figure 2.1).

The use of the water-hardening variety of cements is desirable for luting because, in this form, hand-mixing is simpler and the initial viscosity is very low. Setting time in the oral cavity is probably a little faster and shelf-life is excellent.

Unlike the zinc phosphate cements, it is not possible with the luting cements to vary the setting time to any extent. With the former, chilling the slab and adding the powder in small increments gives the clinician some degree of control of working and setting times. However, the viscosity is somewhat higher in the first place, and it is necessary to maintain positive pressure after placement to ensure that the appliance does not lift off the tooth before the cement is set. Under these circumstances, venting a crown is desirable.

With the glass-ionomer cements, there is a rapid snap set, whether the slab is chilled or not and regardless of the rate at which the powder is incorporated into the liquid. Increase in viscosity and achievement of a snap set varies between products, and the anhydrous types tend to allow longer working time before becoming too viscous to permit full placement of the restoration (Figures 2.3, 2.4). In addition, the cement flows so readily that the appliance does not need to be held under pressure during setting.

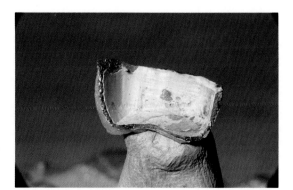

Figure 2.1

A porcelain-bonded-to-metal crown which was removed about 2 years after placement because of loss of porcelain. It has been cut in two to show the cement still attached to the gold rather than to the tooth. Note also the even layer of cement over the entire surface, although the crown was not vented.

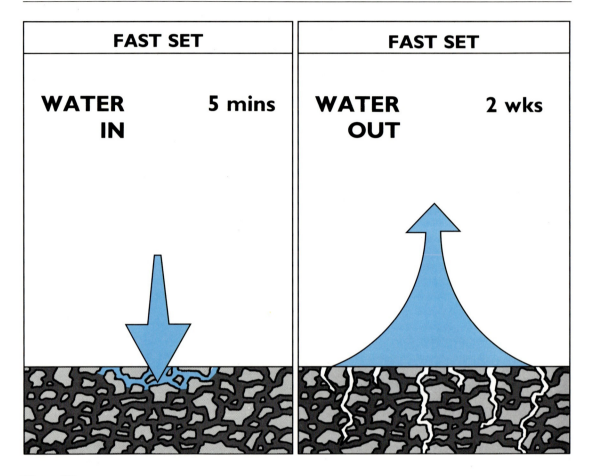

Figure 2.2

Diagram showing the water balance of the Type I glass-ionomer cements. Note that they are resistant to water uptake within about 5 minutes of the start of mix, but remain subject to water loss for about 2 weeks after placement.

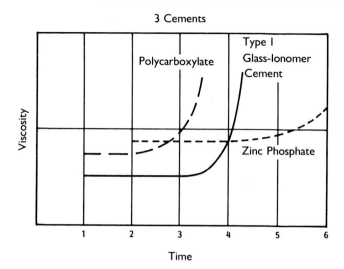

Figure 2.3

Comparison of development of viscosity of freshly-mixed cements and ability to allow complete seating. Note that zinc phosphate cement is initially more viscous but allows seating for longer than the glass-ionomers. Adapted from Øilo and Evje, 1986.

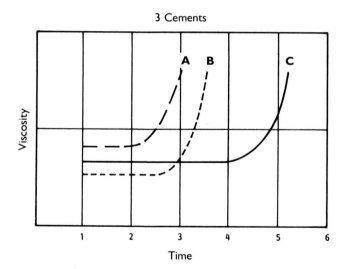

Figure 2.4

Rapid development of viscosity in glass-ionomer cements. All glass-ionomer cements tend to a 'snap' set once the viscosity begins to rise, so working time is not great. Adapted from Øilo and Evje, 1986.

A   Anhydrous cement, using dehydrated poly(acrylic acid) in the powder and water as the liquid
B   Standard cement, using poly(acrylic acid) as the liquid
C   Anhydrous cement, using dehydrated poly(maleic acid) in the powder and dilute tartaric acid as the liquid

Significant factors

Powder/liquid ratio

Powder/liquid ratio is generally about 1.5:1. A moderate increase in powder content is acceptable, although this may reduce the working time and, if increased too far, will give unacceptable ultimate film thickness. Dispensing in capsules and machine mixing is the best method of control and will ensure standard repeatable results. If mixing is to be carried out by hand-working, time can be extended to a limited extent by chilling the slab and the powder – but not the liquid – to a temperature just above the dew point.

Time to mature

Under many circumstances, the gingival margin of a restoration will be sub-gingival and so impossible to isolate during cementation. It is therefore desirable for luting cements to be fast-setting and to have high resistance to water contamination within 5 minutes of the start of mix. It is then unnecessary to seal the cement under a waterproof varnish or resin bond. It should be noted, however, that the cements remain subject to dehydration if left isolated for longer than 10 minutes from the start of mix. This means that water balance must be maintained by releasing the cement to the oral environment within that time.

Adhesion to enamel and dentine

It is possible to develop chemical adhesion to dentine and enamel, and it is also possible to gain a degree of adhesion to noble metals by coating the fitting surface of the restoration with a 2–5 μ layer of tin oxide. Of course, for restorations constructed by an indirect technique retention should be derived from the design of the preparation and the fine fit of the restoration. The luting cement should be present only to seal the interface between restoration and tooth, and should not be relied upon to provide adhesion.

Cementation on vital teeth

In cementation of a full crown, it is possible to develop considerable hydraulic pressure, so it is undesirable to open up dentinal tubules to any degree at all. Therefore, conditioning the surface of the dentine and removing the smear layer with mild acids, such as 10 per cent poly(acrylic acid), is contraindicated. If preparation of the dentine is desired, then a solution such as Causton's ITS solution (see page 19) or 25 per cent tannic acid should be applied for approximately 2 minutes prior to cementation. Either of these will seal the smear layer onto the surface and cover dentinal tubules.

Cementation on non-vital teeth

If the restoration is being placed on a non-vital tooth, development of optimum adhesion is possible. The remaining tooth structure should be conditioned with an application of 10 per cent poly(acrylic acid) for 10–15 seconds to remove the smear layer, washed thoroughly and then dried with a light application of alcohol. The dentine should then be dried but not dehydrated and the cement applied without further contamination.

Fluoride release

Fluoride release is available but, in the light of the small quantity of cement present at the margin, it cannot be relied upon for remineralization of adjacent and surrounding tooth structure.

Pulp compatibility

There has been some controversy concerning possible adverse pulp response and post-insertion sensitivity when using some cements in this group. However, there is a high degree of compatibility between the cement and the pulp under normal circumstances, and the dentine is in itself a very efficient buffer against variations in pH levels.

Recent surveys suggest that the incidence of sensitivity is not, in fact, greatly at variance with other cements, such as the zinc phosphate group. Generation of hydraulic pressure may complicate the response if the dentinal tubules have been opened up by removal of the smear layer. Therefore, a vital tooth should not be conditioned prior to cementation. Alternatively, the surface may be sealed with Causton's ITS solution or 25 per cent tannic acid for 2 minutes. Venting of full crowns is a further precaution which may assist in avoiding problems.

Physical properties

The physical properties have been shown to be equivalent to, or better than, the zinc phosphate cements, and the glass-ionomer cements are becoming the standard against which other cements are measured. Solubility is low, provided that the powder/liquid ratio is high enough, and compressive and tensile strength is adequate, because of the fine particle size.

Radiopacity is desirable so that cement residue can be detected in areas of difficult access.

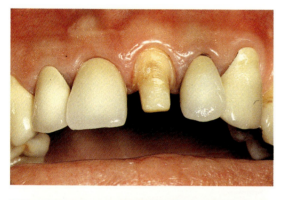

Clinical application

Vital tooth

Figure 2.5

Cementation of a crown for an upper-left central incisor. The temporary crown has been removed and the preparation cleaned ready for cementation.

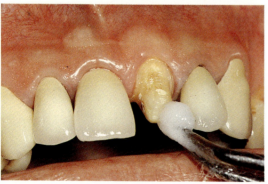

Figure 2.6

The exposed dentine is painted with Causton's ITS solution for 2 minutes and then washed and dried, but not dehydrated.

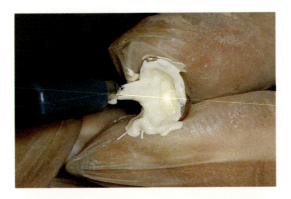

Figure 2.7

Cement is mixed as required and painted on to the fitting surface of the crown with a small, stiff-bristle brush.

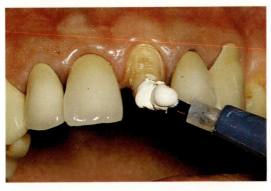

Figure 2.8

A little cement is painted onto the prepared tooth as well.

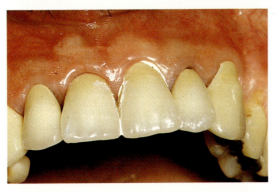

Figure 2.9

The crown is positioned fully in place. A wooden spatula can be used if necessary, but there is no need to maintain pressure.

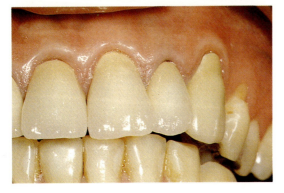

Figure 2.10

The finished crown about 6 months after cementation.

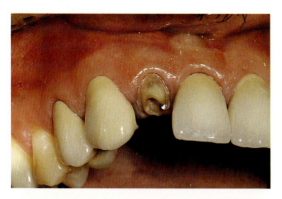

Non-vital tooth

Figure 2.11

Cementation of a post and crown on an upper-right lateral incisor. The temporary crown and post have been removed and the preparation cleaned.

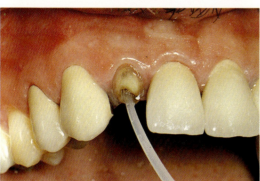

Figure 2.12

The root face and posthole are conditioned with 10 per cent poly(acrylic acid) for 15 seconds to remove the smear layer and enhance retention.

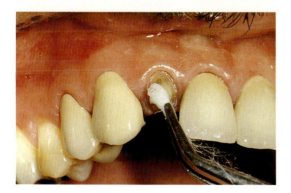

Figure 2.13

The area is washed thoroughly and dried with alcohol, paying particular attention to the apical end of the posthole.

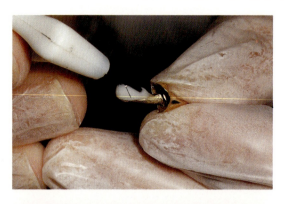

Figure 2.14

Cement is mixed as required and a little painted onto the post.

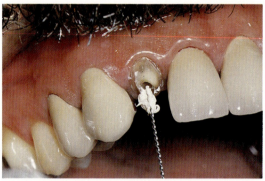

Figure 2.15

Cement is wound into the posthole using an engine-driven Lentulo spiral or similar. The canal is filled to the top.

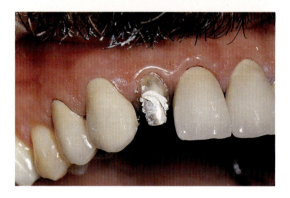

Figure 2.16

The post is positioned and adequate pressure applied to seat it using a wooden spatula. There is no need to maintain pressure.

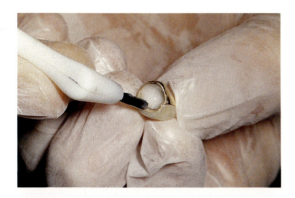

Figure 2.17

The inside of the crown is painted with cement using a small, stiff-bristle brush.

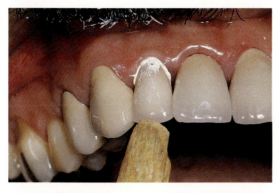

Figure 2.18

The crown is positioned and pressure applied with a wooden spatula. There is no need to maintain pressure.

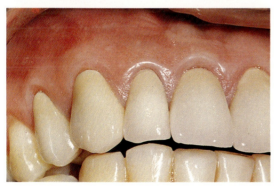

Figure 2.19

The finished crown about 6 months after cementation.

3

Type II.1: Restorative aesthetic cements

Description

Restorative aesthetic cements are the original glass-ionomer cements and the type which has caused the most problems and controversy. An unfortunate tendency has developed in recent years to look for a restorative material that can be contoured and polished completely at the one appointment. For a number of reasons this would appear to be undesirable. If occlusal surfaces are involved, then a reassessment of the occlusion is generally necessary. If the restoration is meant to be aesthetic, then a further check on colour matching is desirable. Polishing prior to the completion of chemical activity and dimensional change in any restorative material should be avoided, and glass-ionomer cement is no exception to this rule.

The glass-ionomer cements enjoy all the properties of the ideal restorative material except that they lack physical resistance to undue occlusal load. Colour matching can be satisfactory and translucency is available, although it takes a few days to develop (see Figures 1.19, 1.20). Adhesion to both enamel and dentine is available and biocompatibility is of a high order, which means that pulp irritation is not a problem. Fluoride release is a major advantage and there have been no reports of microleakage or recurrent caries. Clinical handling is not particularly demanding and long-term stability in the oral environment has been well proven.

Significant factors

Powder/liquid ratio

Powder/liquid ratio varies among the materials currently available, from approximately 2.5:1 to 3:1, for materials using hydrated poly(alkenoic acid) as the liquid, up to as high as 6.8:1, for one of the anhydrous types. Within limits, the higher powder content leads to optimum physical properties. The translucency of the ultimate restoration is, to a large extent, related to the heat history of the glass during manufacture, as well as to the fluoride concentration. The glass utilized in the restorative cements has a lower fluoride content but, with the addition of tartaric acid in the liquid, the setting time remains clinically acceptable and translucency can be achieved with correct handling. A reduction in the powder content may marginally increase translucency but will, at the same time, reduce physical properties. Conversely, it is possible to increase the powder content to such a degree that not all the particles will be reacted and this, of course, will result in a reduction of translucency.

It is difficult to measure a standard quantity of both powder and liquid when attempting to mix by hand. There will also be incorporation of relatively large porosities during mixing, and placement into the cavity by hand will tend to aggravate the situation. It is possible to mix by hand and transfer the cement to a disposable syringe, but this is rather cumbersome and time-consuming, particularly as working time with these cements is generally relatively short.

Dispensing the powder and the liquid in a capsulated system that converts to a syringe is desirable, as the end result will be standard and predictable. Mixing time is reduced but working time does not alter because there is a slight

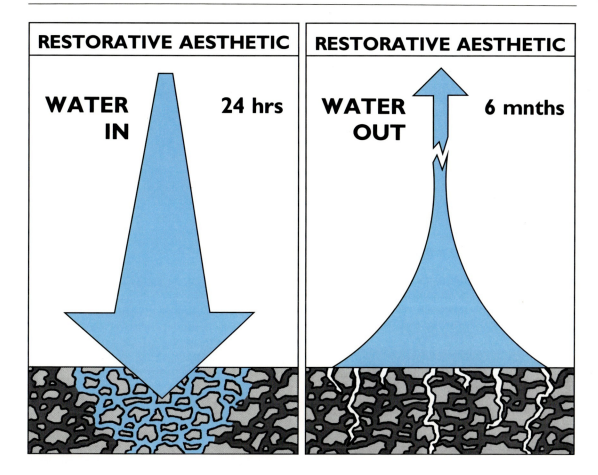

Figure 3.1

Diagram illustrating the water balance of the Type II.1 restorative aesthetic glass-ionomer cements. Note that water uptake is a serious problem in the early stages following placement. Water will penetrate through the entire depth of the cement very rapidly and downgrade both physical properties and, more importantly, translucency. It is also important to be aware of the potential of water loss for up to 6 months after placement.

temperature increase during mixing. This temperature increase tends to encourage a snap set. Placement with a syringe will minimize incorporation of further voids, and the porosities will be relatively small and evenly distributed.

Time to mature

This particular group of glass-ionomer cements remains slow setting, with a prolonged chemical reaction occupying a period of several days, possibly months. This property cannot be altered or speeded up without reducing the translucency.

There is an initial snap set at approximately 4 minutes from the start of mix, at which time it is possible to remove the matrix and examine for successful placement. However, at this point it is extremely susceptible to water uptake and water loss. It is, therefore, essential to keep the cement completely covered with a waterproof sealant for as long as possible to allow full chemical maturation before exposure to the oral environment. It should be painted with the sealant as the matrix is removed.

Manufacturers supply a special varnish as the sealant but, because these varnishes contain an evaporative vehicle, they remain porous to some degree, thus allowing a water exchange both in and out. If these varnishes are to be used, they should be placed in two layers and dried carefully after each application for a period of approximately 30 seconds (see Figure 1.5).

It has been shown that a more effective sealant is a single component, very low viscosity, light-activated, unfilled bonding resin (part of the composite resin system), which has been vacuum packed and is therefore free of porosities (see Figure 1.6). This should be flowed over the restoration in a generous layer immediately the matrix is removed. The restoration can be trimmed as necessary through this layer. When the contour is completed, further resin bond may be added as required and should then be light activated. This will provide a complete seal for at least an hour. Water exchange may occur very slowly over the next 24 hours, at which time the resin sealant can be removed and the restoration

polished under air/water spray. Optimum translucency and physical properties can be obtained using this technique (see Figure 1.14).

The cement should not be challenged with dehydration until up to 6 months after placement. If it is necessary to expose an immature restoration during this period, it should be protected again with a further application of the resin bonding agent or the varnish for the time that it is exposed (see Figure 1.17).

Adhesion to enamel and dentine

Chemical union with underlying tooth structure is one of the greatest advantages with the use of the glass-ionomer cements. It means that an erosion lesion does not need to be instrumented, and a carious cavity does not require the traditional mechanical undercut design for retention. There will be no microleakage and, in conjunction with the fluoride release, there will be almost total prevention of recurrent caries.

The smear layer and other surface contaminants left following cavity preparation should be removed with a 15-second application of 10 per cent poly(acrylic acid). The area should be washed thoroughly with air/water spray. The tooth should be dried gently, but not dehydrated, and the cement placed immediately.

For the erosion/abrasion lesion where no cavity preparation has been undertaken, it is desirable to remove any plaque or pellicle first by lightly scrubbing with a slurry of pumice and water for 5 seconds. This should be washed off and the area lightly dried. The poly(acrylic acid) is then applied for 15 seconds before washing and drying again. The resultant surface will be completely free of contaminants and in a condition to accept chemical union between the restorative cement and the tooth.

Fluoride release

Following successful placement and polishing of the glass-ionomer cement, there will be a high rate of fluoride release for a period of 12–18 weeks thereafter, which can be traced into surrounding and adjacent tooth structure. Although the rate of release will then decline, it has been measured as continuing at a steady level for a further 24 months and probably longer. In the presence of professional or home-applied topical applications of fluoride, and routine use of a fluoride-containing toothpaste, a fluoride balance will develop with the cement, and a continual flow can be predicted.

There is a notable lack of plaque accumulation on glass-ionomer cement restorations, at least in part because of the fluoride release, and tissue tolerance is therefore high (see Figure 1.36).

Pulp compatibility

Pulp tolerance to the glass-ionomer cements has been reported by several authors to be very high, and clinical results substantiate this (Wilson and McLean, 1988). Dentine is a very efficient buffer in itself and the large, complex molecular chains of calcium and aluminium polyacrylate cannot penetrate to any great depth. Nevertheless, if there appears to be less than 0.5 mm of dentine remaining over the pulp chamber, it is suggested that a small quantity of fast-setting calcium hydroxide be placed as protection for the pulp. Note that the minimum of dentine should be covered, because the glass-ionomer cement will only react chemically with the tooth structure and not with the calcium hydroxide (see Figure 1.37).

Physical properties

With the formulations of present glass-ionomer cements, fracture resistance is insufficient to withstand direct occlusal load without adequate support from surrounding tooth structure. Physical properties are largely dependent upon the powder/liquid ratio, so that material which is dispensed in capsule form and is machine mixed will be superior to the hand-mixed materials.

Abrasion resistance and solubility are closely linked with longevity, and are also dependent upon the powder/liquid ratio (see Figure 1.41, 1.42) as well as maintenance of the water balance until full maturity is achieved (see Figure 1.20).

The incorporation of radiopacity tends to alter the colour and translucency so most of this group of cements are radiolucent. However, there are some cements on the market in which a compromise has been achieved, and these can be used for tunnels and Class I/fissure seals where good colour is useful, but not paramount, and radiopacity is desirable.

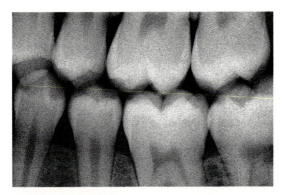

Clinical application

Class I/fissure seal

Figure 3.2

Bitewing radiograph showing a carious lesion under the distal pit on the occlusal surface of the lower first molar (patient aged 18 years).

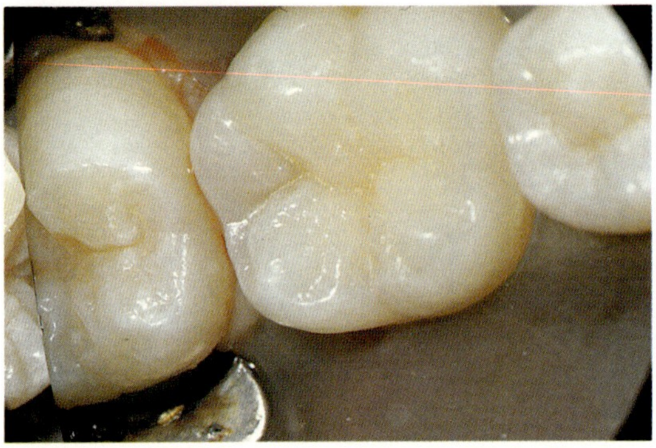

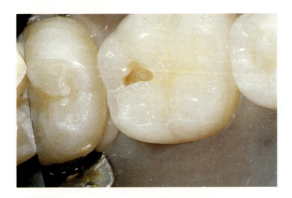

Figure 3.3

Occlusal view of the tooth shown in the radiograph. Note the subtle change of colour under the distal pit, suggesting that there may be caries present.

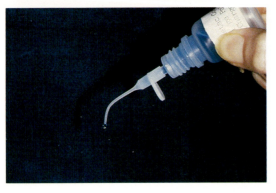

Figure 3.4

Enamel has been removed over the carious lesion disclosing the extent of the problem. If there is any doubt, open the remaining fissures slightly using a very fine diamond stone, without penetrating through the enamel unless the presence of caries dictates it.

Figure 3.5

On completing the cavity, 10 per cent poly(acrylic acid) is applied for 10 seconds, then washed thoroughly with air/water spray.

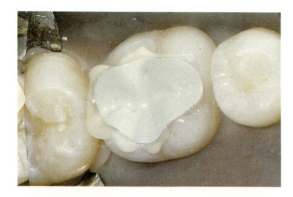

Figure 3.6

To obtain a completely aesthetic restoration and fissure seal, a Type II.1 restorative aesthetic cement can be used – possibly with a degree of radiopacity. The matrix here is a Hawe no 723 which has been preformed to the occlusal surface.

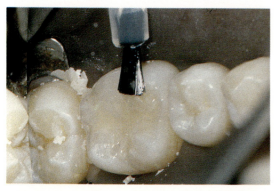

Figure 3.7

As soon as the cement has set, the excess is cleared from around the matrix, the matrix removed and the area immediately painted with a low-viscosity, light-activated bonding resin. The cement is trimmed as required through the unset resin. Further resin is added as necessary, and light activated prior to removing the rubber dam or cotton rolls and releasing the restoration to the oral environment.

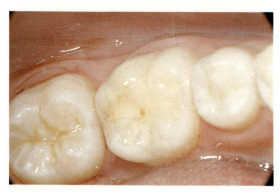

Figure 3.8

The finished restoration, 1 week after placement.

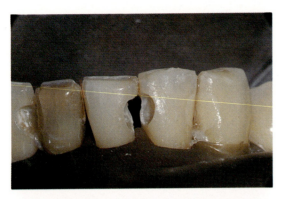

Class III restoration

Figure 3.9

Distal Class III cavity in the lower-left central incisor, and a mesial Class III in the adjacent lateral incisor. Old composite resins which were leaking at the gingival margins have been removed and these dictate the size and design of the cavities.

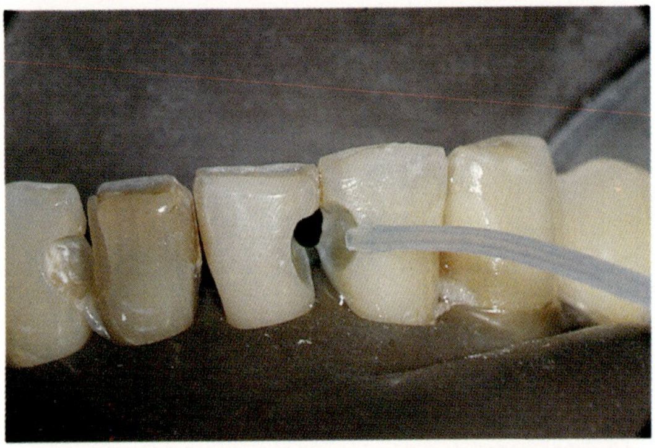

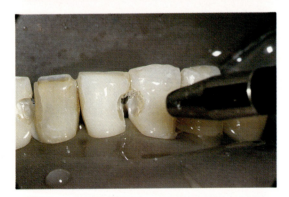

Figure 3.10

Having ensured that the pulp is not exposed, the cavities are conditioned with 10 per cent poly(acrylic acid) for 15 seconds.

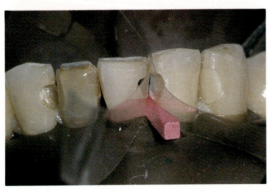

Figure 3.11

At 15 seconds, the cavities are washed thoroughly with air/water spray and dried, but not dehydrated.

Figure 3.12

Mylar strips are used as matrices and wedged positively at the gingival margin to ensure good contour.

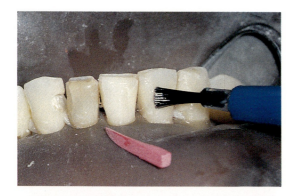

Figure 3.13

Immediately the initial set is achieved, the matrices are removed and the restoration painted with a generous layer of a low-viscosity, light-activated bonding resin. The excess cement is trimmed through the unset resin until the contour is satisfactory. Resin is reapplied as necessary.

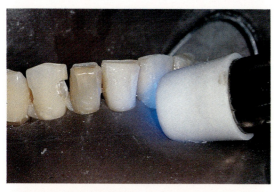

Figure 3.14

The resin is light activated for 10 seconds from both sides.

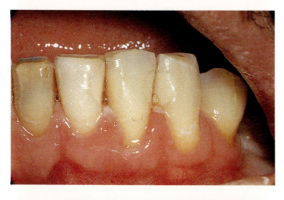

Figure 3.15

Appearance immediately after the removal of the rubber dam.

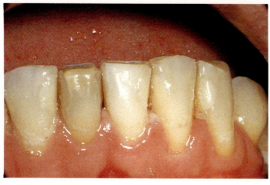

Figure 3.16

Appearance approximately 3 weeks after insertion.

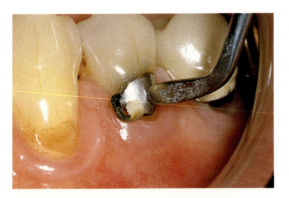

Class V carious cavity

Figure 3.17

Old amalgam restoration on the buccal of the lower-left first bicuspid which appeared to be standing out from the cavity slightly. On the application of firm pressure, plaque was extruded from the mesial margin. As the amalgam was about to be lost, it was decided to replace it with glass-ionomer cement.

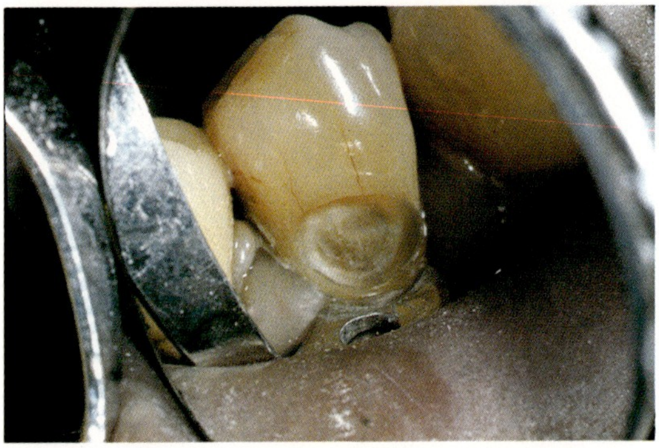

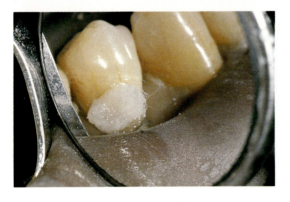

Figure 3.18

The old amalgam has been removed from the cavity and all remaining plaque and demineralized dentine has been removed.

Figure 3.19

The prepared cavity is now conditioned with 10 per cent poly(acrylic acid) for 15 seconds, then washed thoroughly with air/water spray and dried but not dehydrated.

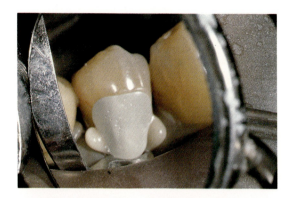

Figure 3.20

The cement is syringed into place and the matrix applied and left undisturbed for 4 minutes from the start of mix. The matrix is a preformed Hawe no 721.

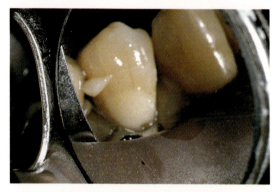

Figure 3.21

The excess cement is removed from around the matrix before lifting the matrix and painting with a generous layer of light-activated unfilled bonding resin. If required the restoration can be trimmed through the unset resin, then further resin added and light activated.

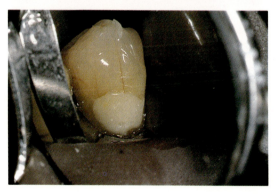

Figure 3.22

The restoration upon completion.

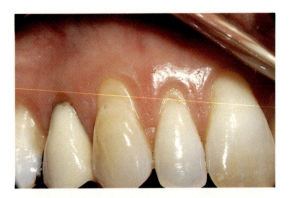

Class V erosion lesion

Figure 3.23

Erosion lesions are present at the gingival margins of the upper-right lateral incisor and canine.

Figure 3.24

Prior to cleaning the teeth, soft-tin matrices (Hawe no 720) are bent to form and tested against the teeth to ensure an accurate fit.

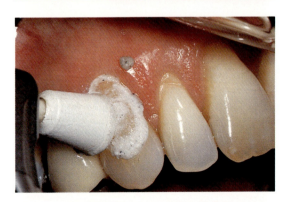

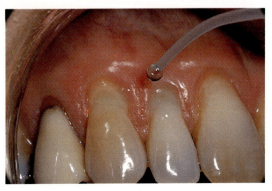

Figure 3.25

The lesions are cleaned with a slurry of pumice and water for 5 seconds only. The pumice is then flushed away and the tooth lightly dried.

Figure 3.26

Ten per cent poly(acrylic acid) can now be applied and left for 15 seconds before washing and drying lightly. Dehydration should be avoided.

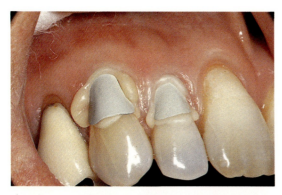

Figure 3.27

The selected shade of cement is now syringed into place and the matrices positioned and left undisturbed while the cement sets. At 4 minutes from the start of mix, the excess cement can be tested for degree of set and then broken away to clear the margins.

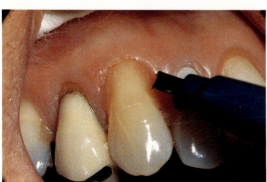

Figure 3.28

Immediately the matrices are removed the cement is covered with a generous layer of an unfilled, light-activated bonding resin. Further trimming can be undertaken and more bond applied if necessary.

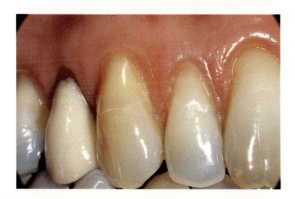

Figure 3.29

The resin is then light activated. Note that there is likely to be a small amount of excess resin at the gingival margin which may act as an overhang. This should be removed with a sharp blade prior to releasing the patient.

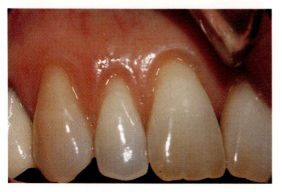

Figure 3.30

The finished restorations, 6 months after placement.

BOX D   TRICHLORACETIC ACID

The profession has a need for efficient methods of haemostasis. Trichloracetic acid is not new but has not been popular or routinely used for some years now. However, it is a very safe and reliable method of controlling haemorrhage in areas of local tissue damage, with virtually no side-effects (see Figures 3.33, 4.19). It is highly caustic but self-limiting and therefore does not penetrate far into soft tissue. The resulting eschar separates from the subjacent tissue without producing an inflammatory response and healing is rapid and uneventful. It will arrest gingival haemorrhage but will remove granulation tissue to a limited extent only.

- Purchase in crystal form.
- Leave the top off the bottle for a few days and the crystals will deliquesce, leaving a liquor of concentrated trichloracetic acid.
- Handle with care.
- When required, dispense 2 or 3 drops with a glass dropper into a Dappen's dish.
- Touch the blade of a no 6 flat plastic instrument or similar into the liquid and convey this to the appropriate place on the soft tissue. Do not apply more than this quantity at any one time. Local anaesthesia is not required.
- The effect will generally be immediate. Repeat if necessary.
- Wash thoroughly with water.

Wolfort FG, Dalton WE, Hoopes JE, Chemical peel with trichloracetic acid, *Brit J Plastic Surg* (1972) **25**: 333–4.

Heithersay GS, Tissue response in the rat to trichloracetic acid – an agent used in the treatment of invasive cervical resorption, *Aust Dent J* (1988) **33**: 451–61.

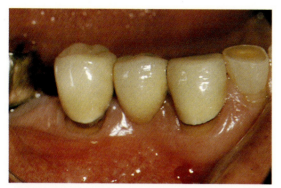

Repair of an existing crown

Figure 3.31

There have been porcelain crowns on the lower-right canine and the second bicuspid as part of a three-unit bridge for approximately 15 years. There are now quite deep erosion lesions at the gingival margins of both abutment teeth. The lesion at the gingival of the second bicuspid extends approximately 2 mm subgingivally, so a minor gingivectomy needs to be carried out.

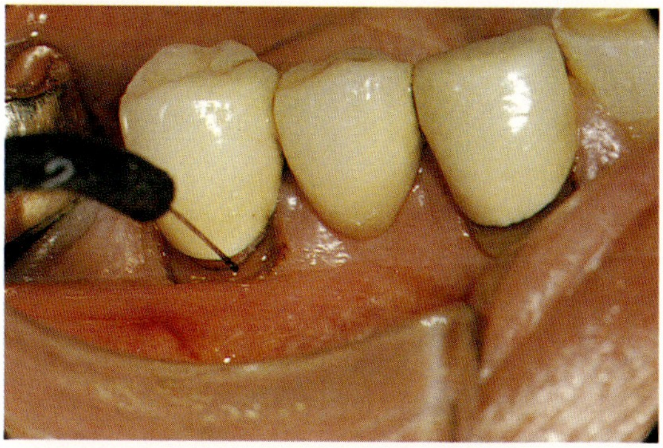

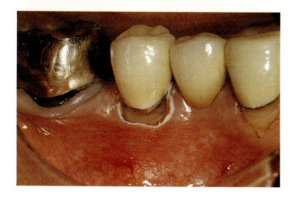

Figure 3.32

Using electrosurgery, approximately 2 mm of gingival tissue is removed to expose the gingival margin of the erosion lesion.

Figure 3.33

As there was a minor amount of haemorrhage in the gingival tissue following electrosurgery, a very light application of trichloracetic acid (see Box D) has been applied to control the haemorrhage. This produces instant haemostasis and will repair readily as the acid is self-limiting.

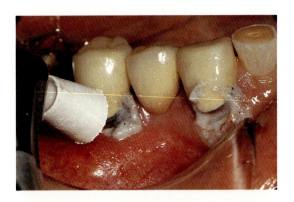

Figure 3.34

Having gained access to both lesions, they are cleaned with a slurry of pumice and water on a rubber cup and washed thoroughly.

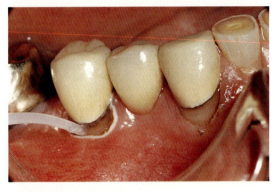

Figure 3.35

The two lesions are lightly dried and then 10 per cent poly(acrylic acid) is applied for 15 seconds. The teeth are washed thoroughly again and dried but not dehydrated.

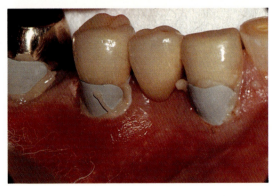

Figure 3.36

Hawe matrices no 721 have been preformed, the cement syringed to place and the matrices adapted to position.

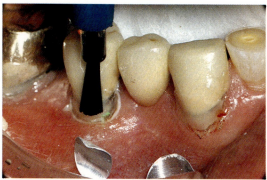

Figure 3.37

At approximately 4 minutes from the start of mix, excess cement can be tested for degree of set and removed prior to lifting the matrices. Immediately the matrices have been removed, a generous layer of a very low viscosity, light-activated resin bonding agent is applied.

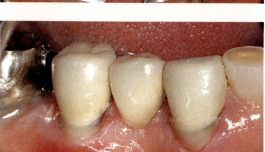

Figure 3.38

The finished restorations 1 week after placement, showing the excellent tissue recovery. There is still an excess contour on both restorations and so they require polishing.

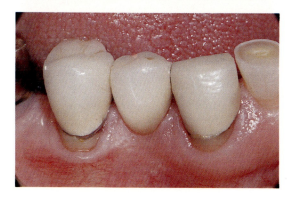

Figure 3.39

The finished restorations, 12 months after placement.

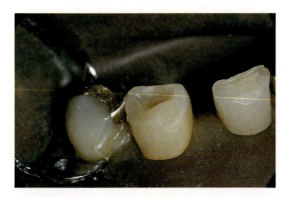

Restoration of an erosion lesion on an incisal edge

Figure 3.40

The incisal edge of the lower-right canine is deeply eroded. However, there is a complete wall of enamel surrounding the entire erosion lesion, so that the glass-ionomer cement will be well supported against lateral and shear stresses.

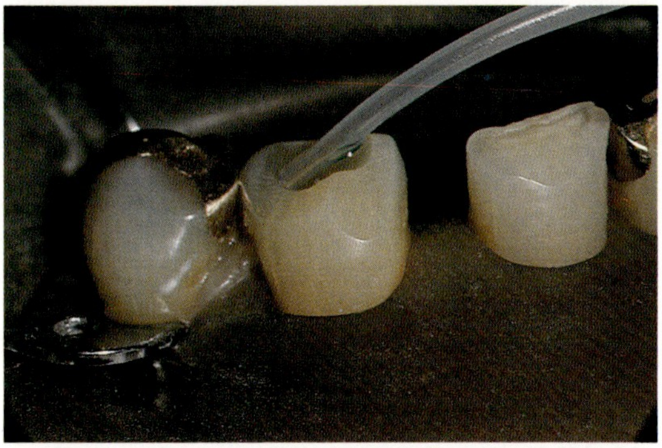

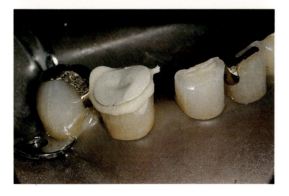

Figure 3.41

Because of the depth of the lesion, it is virtually impossible to scrub with pumice and water, so it is conditioned with 10 per cent poly(acrylic acid) for 15 seconds only. The area is washed thoroughly and dried lightly, but not dehydrated.

Figure 3.42

A Hawe matrix no 722 is preformed, the cement applied and the matrix repositioned.

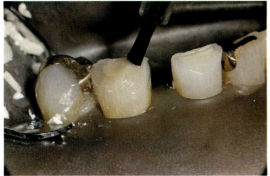

Figure 3.43

At approximately 4 minutes from the start of mix, the excess cement is tested and broken away prior to lifting the matrix. The restoration is immediately covered with a generous layer of very low viscosity, light-activated resin bonding agent. The resin is light activated prior to releasing to the oral environment.

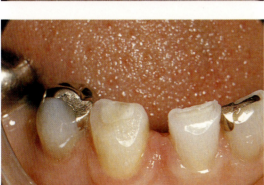

Figure 3.44

Appearance immediately after removal of the rubber dam. The occlusion should be checked and adjusted as required. If the resin bonding agent has been disturbed during adjustment of the occlusion a further layer should be applied before allowing the tooth to get wet.

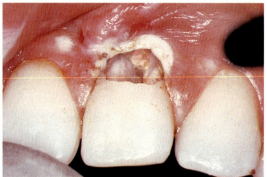

Restoration of an idiopathic external resorption lesion

Figure 3.45

There has been an idiopathic external resorption lesion at the gingival margin of the upper-right central incisor. It extended up under the gingival margin and posed problems for restoration. The resorptive process was dealt with using trichloracetic acid (see Box D, page 46), and the gingival tissue was retracted at the same time.

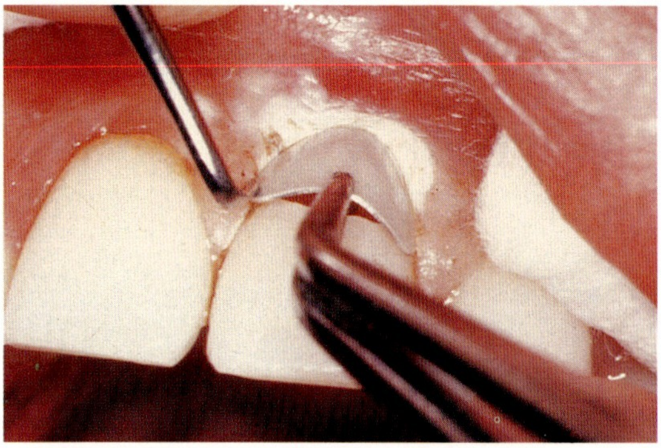

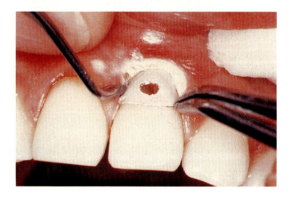

Figure 3.46

A Hawe matrix was preformed to fit the lesion and the cavity was conditioned with 10 per cent poly(acrylic acid) for 15 seconds.

Figure 3.47

The matrix was perforated with a round bur, making a hole in the centre large enough to accept the tip of the nozzle of a capsule. It was then positioned over the lesion.

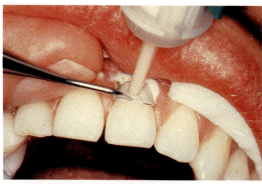

Figure 3.48

The cement was mixed and syringed through the hole until the excess appeared around the periphery of the matrix.

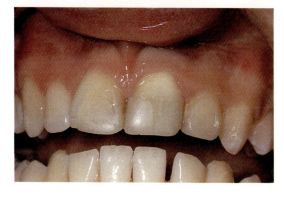

Figure 3.49

The restoration, 2 years after placement, showing complete recovery of the soft tissue.

4 Type II.2: Restorative reinforced cements

Description

As already noted, glass-ionomer cements generally lack fracture resistance and this limits their application in the oral cavity. To date, two different attempts have been made to improve physical properties, but neither has been completely successful. Firstly, there is the so-called 'silver cermet', which is manufactured by incorporating approximately 40 per cent by weight of microfine silver particles, which are sintered to the powdered glass particles. This combination shows improved abrasion resistance to the extent that in this property it compares well with amalgam and composite resin. Compressive strength and fracture resistance are also improved, but not to the extent that it is possible to rebuild cusps and large lesions. Adhesion to dentine and enamel may be slightly reduced because of the presence of the silver particles. In spite of these limitations, the cement has many uses because of its fast set and rapid resistance to water uptake, as well as its radiopacity. It has been advocated for such diverse tasks as Class I restorations, tunnels, core build-ups before crown preparations and many repair situations where the existing restoration is otherwise still fully effective. However, in its present form it is not a universal restorative cement.

Secondly, spherical amalgam alloy powder has been included within a normal Type II restorative aesthetic cement. Physical properties are not significantly improved and, although setting time appears to be enhanced, its resistance to water uptake is not altered. It is radiopaque, but it is so dark in colour that it must always be covered or veneered with another restorative material to be clinically acceptable. Discussion will be limited to the silver-sintered cement.

Significant factors

Powder/liquid ratio

In most clinical situations, optimum physical properties will be required when utilizing this material, so the powder/liquid ratio is important. It is dispensed by the manufacturer in capsule form at the standard ratio of 4:1 but is also available for hand-mixing. Because working time is rather short at the optimum powder/liquid ratio, there is a temptation when hand-mixing to reduce the powder content. This will reduce physical properties and is therefore undesirable. The capsulated version is the material of choice. Also the thick consistency and rather sticky nature of the cement is such that placement with a syringe is desirable. It is possible to use a disposable Centrix type syringe if hand-mixing, but the capsules convert to a syringe and this is the most convenient technique.

Time to mature

This is a fast-setting cement with adequate resistance to water uptake at 5 minutes from the start of mix, and therefore it does not require any protective covering over it as long as it is to be exposed to a humid environment on completion. It can, in fact, be contoured and polished to a complete finish under air/water spray from about 6 minutes from the start of mix. However, it is still not resistant to water loss and remains subject to dehydration, cracking and crazing, for at least 2 weeks after placement. If the newly-placed restoration is to be left exposed for any length of time, or re-exposed in the following 2 weeks while other work is carried out, it should be protected with a layer of low-viscosity, light-activated bonding resin to maintain its water balance.

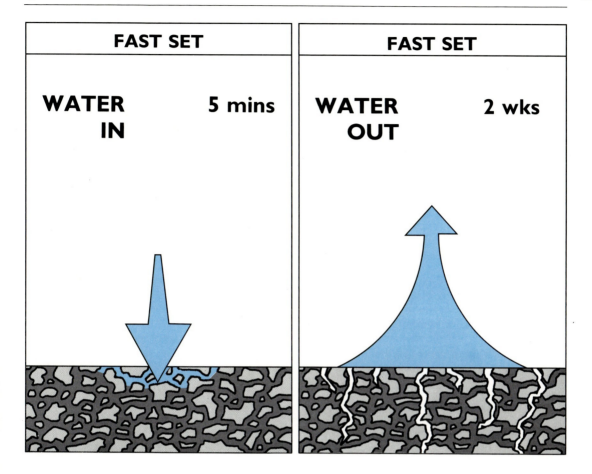

Figure 4.1

Diagram showing the water balance of the Type II.2 glass-ionomer cements. As they are fast setting they are resistant to water uptake in about 5 minutes from the start of mix. This means that they can be polished shortly after removing the matrix. However, if they are left exposed to air for any length of time in the first 2 weeks, they are liable to lose water and crack.

Adhesion to enamel and dentine

The presence of the fine particles of powdered silver sintered to the surface of the glass particles appears to reduce the amount of chemical adhesion available. It is therefore desirable to include a small degree of positive mechanical retention within the cavity design. Conditioning of the surface with 10 per cent poly(acrylic acid) for 15 seconds will remove both the smear layer and other surface contaminants, and will ensure optimum chemical union with the underlying tooth structure.

Fluoride release

Fluoride release seems to be similar to other types of glass-ionomer cement, in spite of the presence of the silver particles. This makes the material particularly suitable for restoring such lesions as root-surface caries and tunnels, where cavity outline is often difficult to determine and remineralization of surrounding tooth structure is important.

Pulp compatibility

Although very little work has been carried out directly on this material, it appears to be just as compatible as the other types of glass-ionomer cement. Direct contact with exposed pulp is contraindicated and, if there appears to be less than 0.5 mm of remaining dentine, a small amount of calcium hydroxide should be placed over the pulp. However, when restoring a lesion, such as root-surface caries, the presence of a peripheral seal eliminating marginal percolation and microleakage means that total removal of softened dentine from the floor of the cavity is not essential.

Physical properties

Both tensile strength and fracture resistance are comparable with the best of the Type II restorative aesthetic cements, but it is still necessary to have the cement well supported by remaining tooth structure (Figure 4.30). Abrasion resistance is improved by the presence of the fine silver particles to such a degree that it is comparable with amalgam and the best of the composite resins in this property. It is theorized that the silver particles allow a degree of slip or flow on the surface.

Because of the presence of the silver, the cement has a radiopacity similar to amalgam. It is therefore possible to reassess marginal integrity and the presence of recurrent caries at a later date.

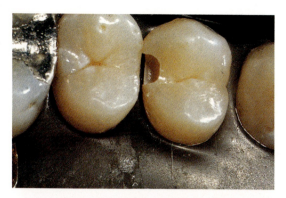

Clinical application

Minimal Class II cavity

Figure 4.2

A very small lesion on the distal of an upper-right first bicuspid. The marginal ridge was already cracked, so a proximal box has been prepared, but the occlusal groove has not been included.

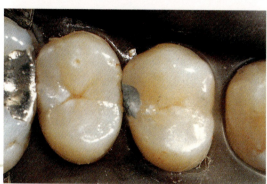

Figure 4.3

The finished restoration after polishing at the insertion appointment.

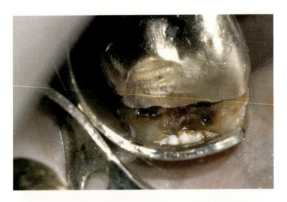

Repair of a crown margin

Figure 4.4

Root-surface caries beyond the gingival margin of a gold crown on a lower-right molar.

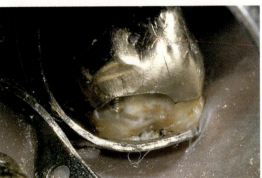

Figure 4.5

The caries has been removed and a limited amount of retention has been placed in the gingival and occlusal wall.

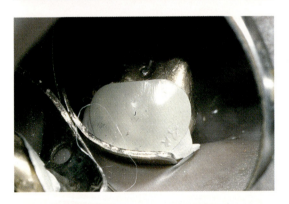

Figure 4.6

The cavity has been conditioned with 10 per cent poly(acrylic acid), and the cement has been syringed to place and supported with a matrix.

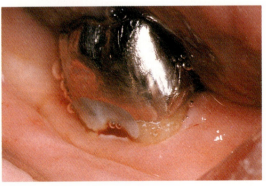

Figure 4.7

Before removal of the rubber dam, the excess cement was trimmed at intermediate high speed under air/water spray. After removal of the dam, the restoration was polished with abrasive rubber points under air/water spray.

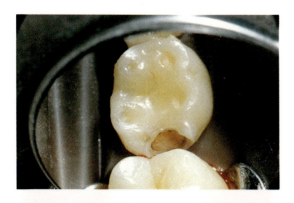

Class II restoration of a deciduous molar

Figure 4.8

A carious lesion on the distal of a deciduous lower molar. The marginal ridge has already been lost.

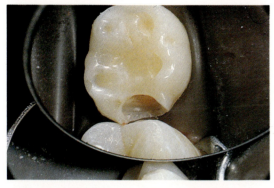

Figure 4.9

The cavity has been cleaned but not extended beyond its original outline. This has allowed maintenance of contact with the adjacent first molar and facilitated the development of a relatively normal contact area during placement of the restoration.

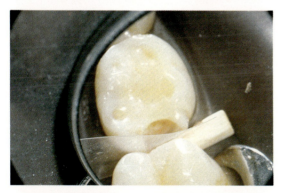

Figure 4.10

A short length of mylar strip has been placed as a matrix and firmly wedged in place.

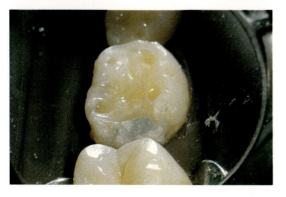

Figure 4.11

The finished restoration which has been polished prior to removal of the rubber dam.

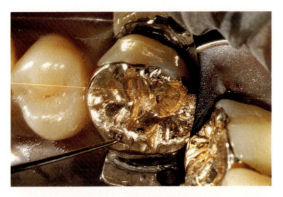

Repair of an inlay margin

Figure 4.12

A small breakdown has been detected on the margin of an otherwise sound gold inlay.

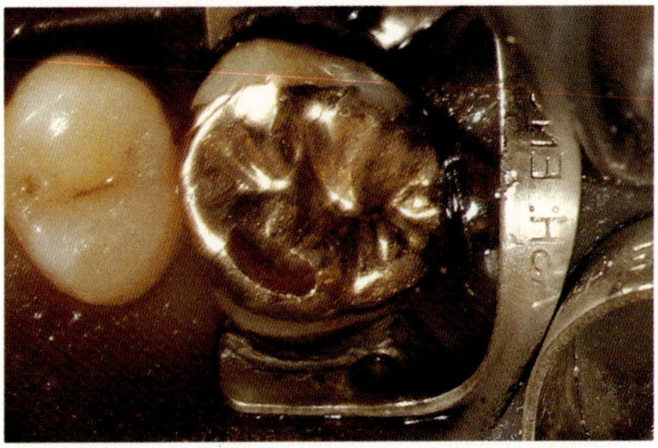

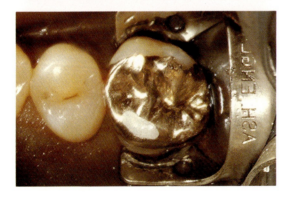

Figure 4.13

The defect has been opened at the expense of both tooth and gold to reveal the extent of the problem. As there is still adequate support for the restoration, glass-ionomer cement is the material of choice.

Figure 4.14

The finished restoration, which has been polished prior to removal of the rubber dam.

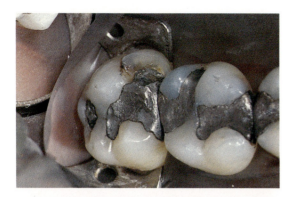

Repair of a broken cusp

Figure 4.15

There has been a limited failure of enamel from the mesio-lingual cusp of an upper molar. As the occlusal load is still borne by the amalgam as well as by the disto-lingual cusp, a minimal cavity was prepared. The amalgam was dressed back and a small amount of retention was included.

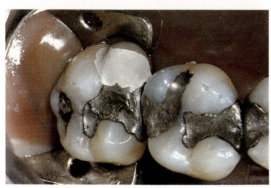

Figure 4.16

The completed restoration.

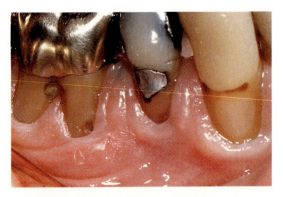

Class V carious cavity

Figure 4.17

This patient demonstrates considerable gingival recession and now displays a series of small root-surface carious lesions. There are two lesions on the buccal of the lower-right first molar, including the furcation area, and a small one on the second bicuspid, beyond the existing amalgam restoration.

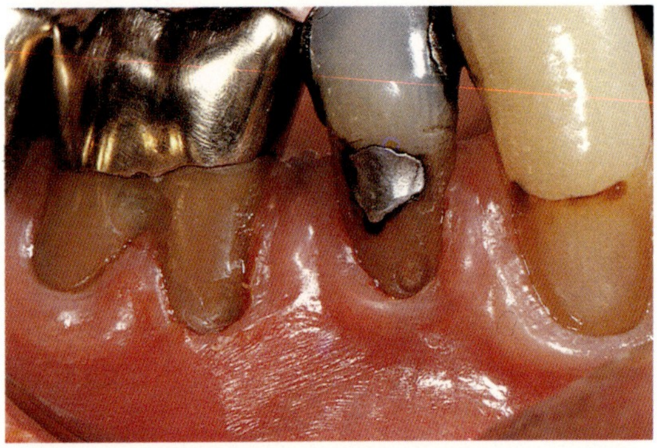

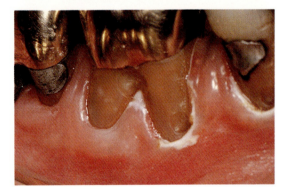

Figure 4.18

Cavities have been prepared, but there is a small amount of damage and thus haemorrhage from the gingival tissues in relation to the two cavities that were partly subgingival.

Figure 4.19

Haemorrhage has been arrested with a limited application of trichloracetic acid (see Box D, page 46), just in the involved areas. As the acid is self-limiting, the tissue will respond and heal readily.

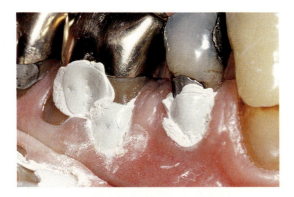

Figure 4.20

Following cavity preparation, the cavities were conditioned with 10 per cent poly(acrylic acid) for 15 seconds, and the teeth were washed thoroughly and dried but not dehydrated. Separate Hawe matrices no 719 were preformed to the three lesions and Ketac Silver was syringed into place.

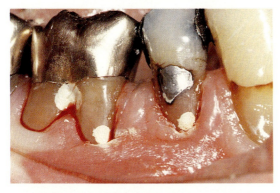

Figure 4.21

At 4 minutes from the start of mix, the excess cement was tested first, then broken away and the matrices removed. At this point the restorations can be contoured and polished to completion under air/water spray, using very fine diamonds and graded rubber polishing cups and points.

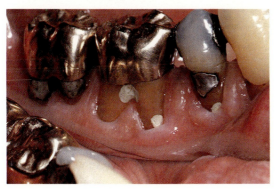

Figure 4.22

The restorations 1 week after placement, showing that the soft tissue has healed completely. The lesion on the second bicuspid, in particular, is already almost submerged into the gingival crevice.

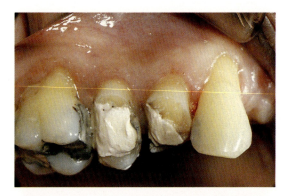

Core build-up for crowns

Figure 4.23

The upper-right first and second bicuspids were both badly broken in a motor vehicle accident. Buccal and lingual cusps were lost from the first bicuspid and buccal cusp only from the second, but both required root-canal treatment.

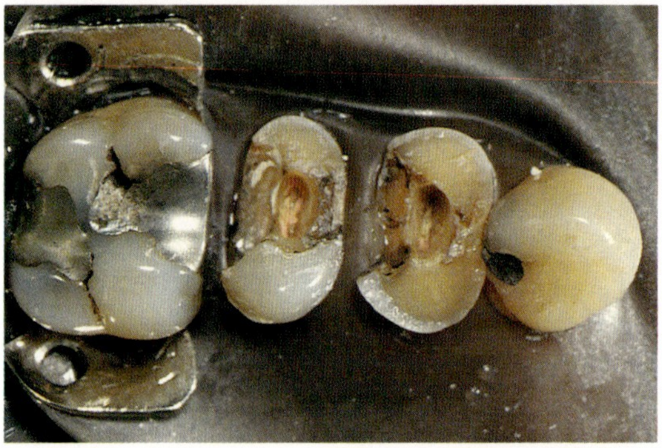

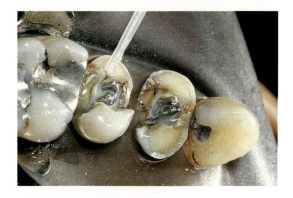

Figure 4.24

The root canals in both teeth have been prepared and the remains of existing restorations removed.

Figure 4.25

Stainless steel posts have been cemented into both teeth. The posts in the first bicuspid protrude beyond remaining tooth structure because it was anticipated that the core would be built-up to that level. The posts in the second bicuspid were cut off to just below the proposed core height because the entire lingual cusp was still present and would provide support. Remaining tooth structure was conditioned with 10 per cent poly(acrylic acid), then washed thoroughly and dried but not dehydrated.

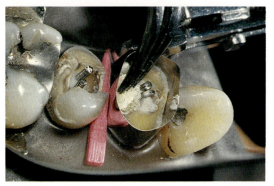

Figure 4.26

A standard steel matrix has been placed on the first bicuspid and Ketac Silver syringed into place incrementally. Each increment was tamped into place with a small plastic sponge (see Figure 7.25) to ensure full adaptation to underlying tooth structure and around the two posts.

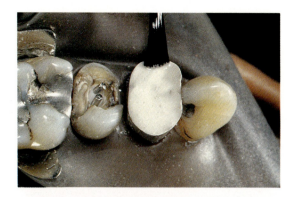
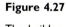

Figure 4.27

The build-up on the first bicuspid is complete and the matrix removed. However, as this was to remain isolated and dry for a period while the second bicuspid was restored in the same way, the freshly-placed Ketac Silver was covered with a generous coating of a very low viscosity, light-activated bonding resin to prevent water loss in the short term.

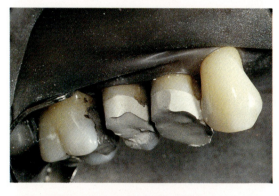

Figure 4.28

The Ketac Silver core has now been built-up on both teeth.

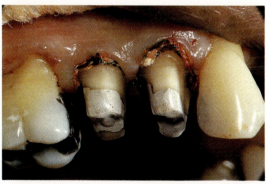

Figure 4.29

A buccal view of the finished crown preparations at the time of gingival retraction. Note that there is at least 2–3 mm of natural tooth structure between the Ketac Silver core and the gingival margin on both teeth, except in relation to the distal proximal boxes.

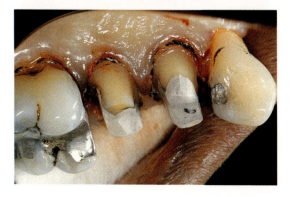

Figure 4.30

A palatal view of the prepared teeth. On the first bicuspid there is at least 3 mm of normal tooth structure between the Ketac Silver and the gingival margin. On the second bicuspid there is the full height of the palatal cusp. This ensures maximum resistance against lateral stresses and minimal load on the Ketac Silver core.

5 Type III: Lining cements

Description

There are a number of cements available which may be broadly described as Type III lining cements. They lack translucency and aesthetics so their use is confined to situations where they are either totally or partially covered by other restorative materials. Their major advantages are: a very fast-setting reaction with early resistance to water uptake; adhesion to dentine and enamel to prevent microleakage; fluoride release; and radiopacity. These properties make them a suitable lining under any restorative material.

A further advantage is that as with all the glass-ionomer cements, Type III lining cements are capable of being etched with 37 per cent orthophosphoric acid, just like enamel and in the same time-span. They are therefore advocated particularly for use as a dentine substitute under composite resin. Following etching, the composite resin can obtain a mechanical interlock to the cement and the so-called 'sandwich restoration' can be constructed. In theory, the cement will attach chemically to the dentine and the composite resin will attach mechanically to the cement and the enamel, thus producing a relatively 'monolithic' structure. Of course, under these circumstances, it is essential to use a high powder/liquid ratio cement in sufficient bulk to be an integral part of the restoration.

Several new restorative techniques have been developed in the last few years for the purpose of avoiding the use of amalgam and gold and improving aesthetics. Both composite resin and porcelain laminate veneer restorations, as well as porcelain inlays, are now being extensively used and protection of and adhesion to dentine is becoming highly significant. It is biologically unacceptable to etch dentine and the present range of dentine-bonding agents appear to have a limited life in the oral environment. All of these techniques utilize a filled or unfilled resin as the bonding agent. Glass-ionomer cement is therefore a valuable intermedi-ary because of its high pulp tolerance, chemical union with the dentine and its ability to be etched and unite mechanically with resin.

The following discussion applies regardless of whether the restoration is placed over the Type III glass-ionomer cement lining, but the more reliance that is placed on the cement, the greater the need for good physical properties. If the cement is being used only as a traditional lining under an amalgam, for example, its physical properties are relatively insignificant. However, if it is to be etched under a composite resin, it should be strong and a minimum of 0.5 mm thick, or it may disintegrate under the influence of the etchant.

The original lining cements are all hand mixed and chemically activated and the powder/liquid ratio can be varied from 1.5 : 1 to 4 : 1, depending on the purpose for which they are being placed. At a low ratio they flow readily and can be easily placed as a traditional lining under other restora-tions such as amalgam and gold. Their early strength is sufficient to withstand the heavy condensation pressures required for the placement of amalgam and they are useful for making up deficiencies and defects in cavities designed for gold or porcelain inlays.

Their ultimate physical properties are however greatly enhanced by increasing the powder/liquid ratio to 4 : 1 or more, when these cements, preferably capsulated for ease of handling, can be regarded as a true dentine substitute. They can then be used as the foundation for such restora-tions as composite resin veneers, porcelain lamin-ates and porcelain inlays.

Their physical properties are such that they can be etched 5 minutes from the start of the mix with 37 per cent orthophosphoric acid, just like enamel and in the same time span. Following etching, the composite resin or resin-bonding agent can pro-duce a mechanical interlock with the cement and the so-called 'sandwich' restoration can be con-structed. In theory the cement will attach chemi-cally to the dentine and the resin will bond

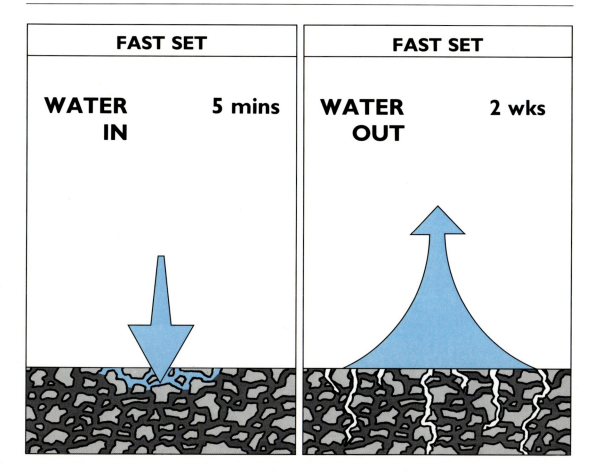

Figure 5.1

Diagram showing the water balance of the Type III glass-ionomer cements. As they are fast setting they are resistant to water uptake in about 5 minutes from the start of mix. This means they can be etched shortly after removing the matrix. However, if they are left exposed to air for any length of time, they are liable to lose water and crack.

mechanically to the cement and enamel, thus producing a relatively monolithic reconstruction of the tooth. Recent work shows that this can return the tooth to as much as 95 per cent of its original strength.

A recent development has resulted in the light-activated glass-ionomer cements and these can also be used as a lining material. At present they are manufactured as a low powder/liquid ratio lining cement only, which should be completely covered with another restoration. The set cement consists of approximately 10 per cent light-activated resin and takes up to 24 hours to achieve its full physical properties. It sets firm under the influence of the light activator but the polyacrylic chains continue to form and the cement is not properly hard for some time. This means that the cement may be damaged during condensation of the amalgam. It

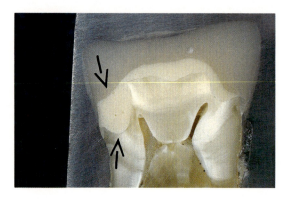

Figure 5.2

A cross-section through a molar tooth showing a simulated design for a 'sandwich' restoration using a cement with a powder/liquid ratio of 3:1. In one proximal box, there is no enamel at the gingival margin. The cement therefore has been built up just short of the contact area and will be left exposed in the oral cavity. At the other end, there is sufficient enamel to bevel and etch, so that the cement remains short of the margin and the union is composite resin to enamel. Note the thickness of cement over the entire cavity floor.

could also be disturbed by the stresses imposed by the setting contraction of composite resin. However, providing the cement is not exposed to the oral environment at the cavity margin, it represents a fast method of placing a lining. Owing to the presence of the resin in the cement, it will attach readily to a composite resin placed over it and it is not necessary to etch it. Similarly, if the lining is to be completely covered with another restoration, chemical attachment to the dentine is unnecessary. Thus conditioning of the cavity is not needed. At the same time, any fluoride release will be confined to the dentine immediately under the cement and will not be available to adjacent teeth.

It must be noted that there have been a number of lining cements placed on the market lately under the title 'glass-ionomer cements' which do not contain poly(alkenoic acid) and therefore do not fit into this category. They consist of a light-activated resin with a high-fluoride glass as the filler, similar to the light-activated calcium hydroxides. While they are satisfactory linings they will not chelate with dentine or release fluoride and, of course, they should not be exposed to the oral environment.

Significant factors

Powder/liquid ratio

The physical properties of these cements are dependent upon the powder/liquid ratio, so that if high strengths are required in the ultimate lining, such as in the 'sandwich' technique, a high powder/liquid ratio, of at least 3:1, must be used. The higher the powder content, the shorter will be both the mixing time and the working time. While most of the lining cements are marketed for hand-mixing, the capsulated varieties, which can be machine mixed, will provide more reliable results with higher physical properties because of the higher powder content.

Cements with a low powder/liquid ratio, in the range of 1.5:1, are useful as all-purpose cavity linings. In thin section, their tensile strength will not be high, but the rapid-setting reaction means early achievement of a compressive strength high enough to withstand the heavy packing pressure used in the placement of amalgam. At this consistency, they are also useful for correcting minor deficiencies when carrying out crown preparation. For correcting major defects, the heavier 3:1 ratio should be used.

Time to mature

All the cements in this group are designed to be resistant to water uptake approximately 5 minutes from the start of mix. They should undergo a snap set at that point, and a final restoration can be placed. Alternatively, they can be lightly cut back and etched ready for the 'sandwich' technique.

Not all cements commercially available at the present time are acceptable for the sandwich technique. Some cements pass through a rubbery phase between 5 and 10 minutes after the beginning of mix and do not set really hard. They appear to be susceptible to water uptake and tend to expand for a period of days after mixing. A test specimen of the cement should be made and if it

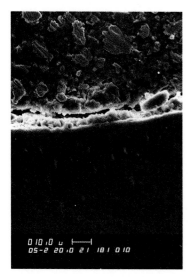

```
0 10 10 u |——|
05-2 20 10 21 18 1 0 10
```

Figure 5.3

SEM showing the ion-exchange layer which is formed between the dentine and cement. Note that failure has occurred in the cement due to dehydration while preparing the specimen for viewing, but the ion-exchange layer stays firmly adherent to the dentine. *Original magnification* x 500.

does not set hard at 7 minutes from the start of mix, it is probably not suitable as a lining.

As with all the glass-ionomers, this group of cements remains susceptible to dehydration for some time after placement. If more than one restoration is being placed in a quadrant, it is wise to place only one lining at a time, and immediately proceed to place the final restoration in that tooth before lining the next. Alternatively, protect the lining with a low-viscosity, light-activated bonding resin or a varnish, to maintain water balance, and remove the cover immediately prior to placing the next restoration.

Adhesion to enamel, dentine and composite resin

Chemical adhesion is available between the cement and underlying tooth structure, provided that the smear layer and other debris has been removed first by conditioning with 10 per cent poly(acrylic acid) for 15 seconds. However, if the cement is being used simply as a conventional lining under an amalgam, for example, then this step is unnecessary and can be omitted (Figures 5.7–5.9).

If the cement is to be used as a base or dentine substitute under composite resin in the 'sandwich' technique, there are two interfaces to be considered (Figure 5.2):

● chemical adhesion between the cement and the dentine
● mechanical union between the cement and the composite resin.

In theory, the technique should work well and provide the optimum 'monolithic' restoration. However, there are some limitations and the following points should be taken into account.

The tensile strength of the cement is the weakest link in the chain. Therefore, the strongest cement available should always be used, particularly if the restoration is to be subjected to heavy occlusal load. The Type III lining cements have been developed with this technique in mind, and the Type II.2 cements are also satisfactory. Some of the Type II.1 restorative aesthetic cements have superior physical properties and better aesthetics, so they are also valuable in the sandwich. Where aesthetics are important, as in a Class IV restoration, the Type II.1 restorative aesthetic cement is the material of choice. However, etching of this cement should be delayed for at least 15 minutes to permit a reasonable advance in maturation before allowing it to get wet. There will be some loss of translucency, but this will be compensated by the composite resin.

The dentine should be conditioned with a 15-second application of 10 per cent poly(acrylic acid) to remove the smear layer and any other contaminants that may be present. This will also pre-activate the calcium ions in the dentine in preparation for the ionic exchange with the cement (Figure 5.3).

The cement must cover all dentine tubules, should never be less than 1 mm thick, and the highest powder/liquid ratio available should be utilized. The cement can then be left exposed to the oral environment at the gingival margin of the restoration and full advantage taken of the adhesion

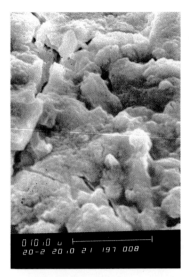

Figure 5.4

SEM of the surface of a glass-ionomer cement which has been cut back after setting but has not yet been etched. Note the matrix investing the glass particles and holding them together. *Original magnification* x 2000.

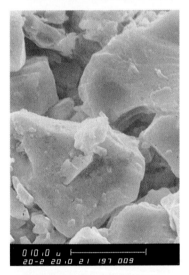

Figure 5.5

SEM of a glass-ionomer cement after etching for 15 seconds with 37 per cent orthophosphoric acid, showing removal of the matrix and development of deep clefts between the particles, into which a low-viscosity resin bonding agent will penetrate. *Original magnification* x 2000.

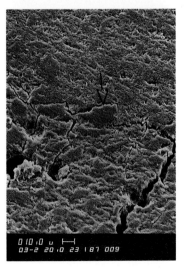

Figure 5.6

SEM of the union between glass-ionomer cement and composite resin. Note the intimate meeting at the interface. The cement is Ketac-fil and the resin is Visio-fil, with VisioBond used as the low-viscosity unfilled resin bonding agent. The crack in the cement is an artefact caused by dehydration of the specimen during preparation for viewing under the SEM. *Original magnification* x 300.

to dentine as well as fluoride release. A cement with a low powder/liquid ratio should not be exposed to the oral environment at the margins of a restoration because its physical properties are not high enough.

Having placed the cement and allowed it to set for 4 minutes, it should be lightly cut back with a fine diamond stone to remove the matrix-rich surface, define the final cavity design and, at the same time, clean and bevel the enamel. Both enamel and cement can now be etched for 15 seconds with 37 per cent orthophosphoric acid and washed thoroughly to remove the etch residue (Figures 5.4, 5.5).

The light-activated glass-ionomer cements do not need to be etched because of the presence of of the resin in the cement, which will bring about union with the composite resin. However, they should not be exposed to the oral environment because solubility, abrasion resistance and adhesion to dentine remain untested so far.

Not all glass-ionomer cements will develop a good etch surface. Generally, those cements which undergo a complete snap set at approximately 4 minutes from the start of mix are acceptable. Some cements currently available achieve an initial set at 4 minutes but then pass through a rubbery phase for a further 10 minutes or thereabouts. These will not etch very effectively, tend to take up further water and later disintegrate, and are therefore undesirable in the sandwich technique.

The chemical action of the etching procedure will develop a high-energy surface on the cement. This will attract a low-energy liquid and result in a very intimate union. Therefore, the unfilled resin bonding agent used to initiate the union between the etched cement and the composite resin should have a very low viscosity so that it will flow easily into the surface voids produced by the etching (Figure 5.6). Some composite resin bonding agents are supplied in two components and contain an evaporative vehicle to reduce viscosity. In clinical use, these generally leave an incomplete film with a degree of porosity which may reduce the effectiveness of the union. Chemically activated bonding agents also show the same problem and are therefore not recommended for this technique.

Composite resins shrink to varying degrees upon polymerization. This dimensional change may exert considerable stress on the union between resin and cement and may result in damage to the cement and loss of union, particularly if either resin or cement has a low tensile strength. The heavily-filled hybrid composite resins generally have a low setting shrinkage and are therefore more acceptable than the lightly-filled microfils, which may show a dimensional change of up to 5 or 6 per cent. Careful incremental build-up is essential to minimize the effect of the dimensional change and to try to ensure that it occurs in the right direction. In addition, the strongest available cement should be used and it should be placed in a substantial layer as a dentine substitute, rather than as a conventional lining.

Fluoride release

Fluoride release is relatively insignificant if the cement is to be entirely covered by another restorative material, such as amalgam or composite resin. However, there are many circumstances in the sandwich technique where the cement will be exposed to the oral environment at the gingival margin, underneath the other material. Fluoride release will then be useful for caries control in both the restored tooth and adjacent ones (Figure 5.2).

Pulp compatibility

If there is less than 0.5 mm of remaining dentine over the pulp chamber, a small discreet area of calcium hydroxide should be laid down to ensure the safety of the pulp. However, dentine itself is a very effective buffer and pulp compatibility appears high, regardless of powder/liquid ratio.

Physical properties

The higher the powder content, the greater the physical properties of the cement, and capsulation will remove all the variables from dispensing. Low powder/liquid ratios are acceptable only when the cement is to be entirely submerged under another restorative material and is not intended to be etched.

The physical properties of the light-activated glass-ionomer cements appear to be acceptable but take some hours to develop. They should not be subjected to undue stress at the time of placement.

All Type III lining cements are radiopaque and, although there is a variation in colour available, none of them is aesthetic or translucent.

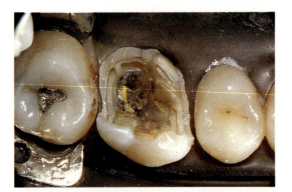

Clinical application

Lining under an amalgam

Figure 5.7

An upper-right first molar with a large cavity present, including the loss of the entire lingual cusps. The radiograph confirms that the pulp has receded and is still vital, and a glass-ionomer lining cement is to be placed. It can be either chemically activated or light activated.

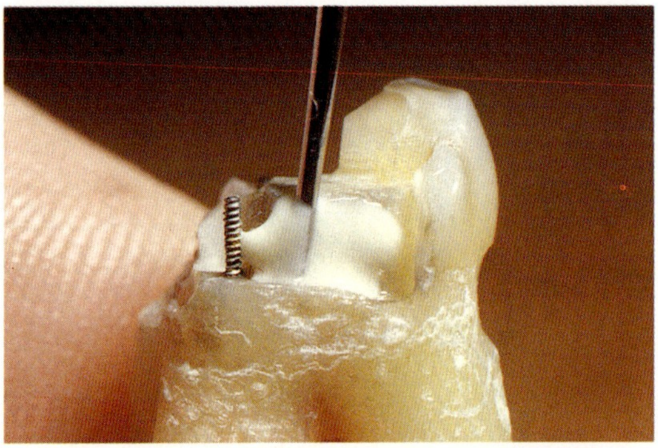

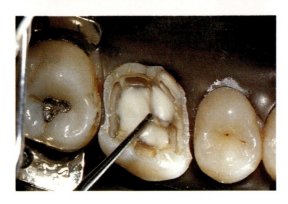

Figure 5.8

As the lining is to be entirely covered by amalgam, there is no need to condition the cavity. The cement will be placed at a powder/liquid ratio of 1.5:1, using a small calcium hydroxide placement instrument to paint the cement lightly over the dentine surface (simulated).

Figure 5.9

The cement placed on the floor of the cavity (Figure 5.7) showing the full extent of the area to be covered. Note that the retention for an amalgam restoration is to be achieved with ditches and grooves.

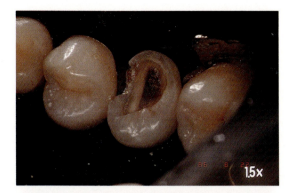

Sandwich technique for a posterior composite resin

Figure 5.10

The upper-left second bicuspid had a large carious lesion beginning in the occlusal fissure and including a small break in the enamel on the mesial proximal surface, so that the entire buccal cusp collapsed. The cavity has been cleaned of all remaining caries and all sound tooth structure has been retained.

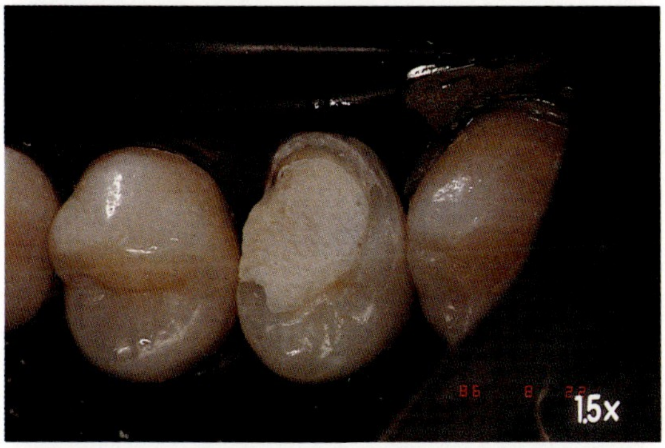

Figure 5.11

After conditioning with 10 per cent poly(acrylic acid) for 15 seconds, the cavity was washed thoroughly and dried but not dehydrated. A mylar strip was placed between the two bicuspids and wedged firmly. Almost the entire cavity was restored with a capsulated Type III glass-ionomer cement at 3:1 powder/liquid ratio and allowed to set for 4 minutes.

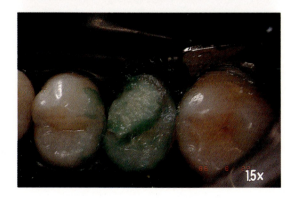

Figure 5.12

Once the cement had set completely, it was cut back with a very fine diamond under air/water spray to remove the matrix-rich surface and expose all available enamel margins. These were cleaned and bevelled. As there was no enamel left at the mesial gingival margin of the proximal box, this was retained entirely in cement.

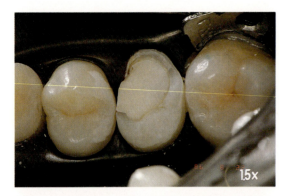

Figure 5.13

Following trimming, contouring and bevelling of the margins, both the cement and the enamel were etched with 37 per cent orthophosphoric acid for 15 seconds. The etchant was thoroughly flushed away and the tooth dried to display the traditional matt finish of etched cement and enamel.

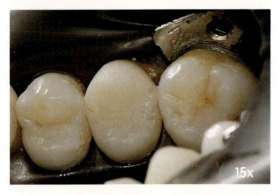

Figure 5.14

The restoration was built up with a hybrid composite resin faced on the buccal with a microfil composite resin.

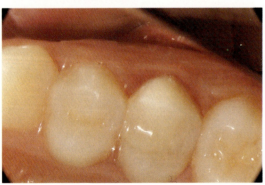

Figure 5.15

The restoration at the 6 month recall.

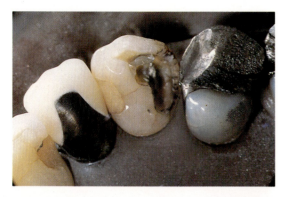

Sandwich technique for an anterior composite resin

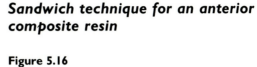

Figure 5.16

The incisal corner has failed over an old Class III amalgam restoration on the distal of the upper-left canine. There is some recurrent caries and the enamel at the gingival is very weak. A glass-ionomer cement/composite resin sandwich is the restoration of choice.

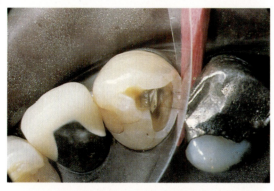

Figure 5.17

The cavity has been cleaned of caries and conditioned with 10 per cent poly(acrylic acid) for 10 seconds and thoroughly washed. A mylar strip has been placed as a matrix and wedged firmly.

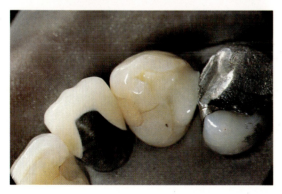

Figure 5.18

As aesthetics is significant for this restoration, a Type II.1 restorative aesthetic cement has been used. Under these circumstances, following initial set, the cement has been covered with a generous layer of a low-viscosity bonding resin and left to mature for 15 minutes after placement.

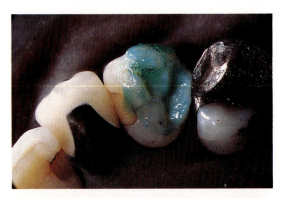

Figure 5.19

At 15 minutes from placement, the cement was lightly cut back under air/water spray to remove the bonding resin, and the matrix-rich surface of the cement and the enamel was bevelled as required. The cement and the enamel were then etched for 15 seconds with 37 per cent orthophosphoric acid.

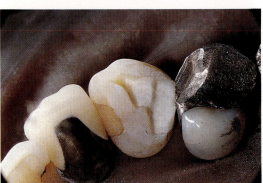

Figure 5.20

The completed cement lining ready for the application of the composite resin. Note that the gingival margin was still covered with a generous layer of cement.

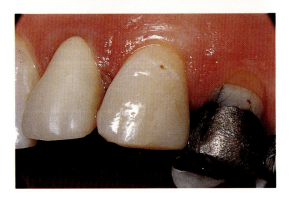

Figure 5.21

The completed restoration after removal of the rubber dam. The glass-ionomer cement extends 2–3 mm from the gingival margin. The aesthetic result justifies the use of the Type II.1 cement.

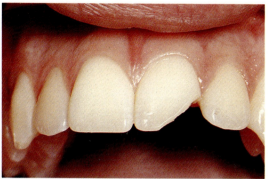

Repair of a traumatized incisal edge

Figure 5.22

Following a motor vehicle accident, this patient presented for emergency treatment with a Class II fracture of the distal incisal corner of the upper-left central incisor. Dentine was exposed but the pulp was still covered and vital.

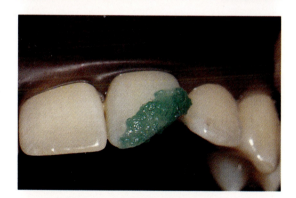

Figure 5.23

The surface was conditioned for 15 seconds with 10 per cent poly(acrylic acid), flushed and lightly dried. A Type II.1 restorative aesthetic cement was syringed over the dentine, without building up the incisal corner. No matrix was used. Prior to complete set of the cement, it was covered with a very low viscosity, light-activated bonding resin to prevent hydration or dehydration. The bond was activated and the patient was immediately comfortable and safe.

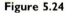

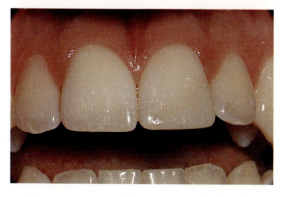

Figure 5.24

Four weeks later, pulp tests suggested that the tooth had settled down and was unlikely to lose vitality, and so it was restored with composite resin. The cement was very lightly cut back to a fresh surface, the enamel was bevelled and both cement and enamel were etched with 37 per cent orthophosphoric acid for 15 seconds. Composite resin was used to build up the corner.

Figure 5.25

The final restoration, photographed at the next 6 month recall visit. Pulp testing showed that the tooth was still vital.

6 Modified cavity designs suitable for restoration with glass-ionomer cements

In treating a carious lesion, dentists are faced with the problem of having to retain as much natural tooth structure as possible, using materials that are relatively difficult to manipulate and that have limited physical properties, making them less than ideal for the purpose. The tooth has already been weakened by the disease process and further loss of enamel or dentine will only exacerbate the situation.

In the past, cavity design has been dictated, to a degree, by the nature of restorative materials available. Amalgam, for example, has to be manually condensed under considerable pressure to adapt it properly to the cavity, to minimize porosities and to eliminate excess mercury. Gold is probably the best restorative material but is expensive and not aesthetic. Much attention has been paid in recent years to composite resin technology and, provided that there is enamel present around the entire margins to provide mechanical adhesion and prevent microleakage, it has several advantages. It is possible to limit destruction of remaining tooth structure and it is aesthetic. However, it is not possible at present to provide long-term adhesion to dentine, its resistance to occlusal load remains an unknown factor and it is very technique-sensitive.

The advent of the glass-ionomer cements has opened up further opportunities to minimize tooth destruction to the extent that, under some circumstances, it is possible to adopt a surgical approach to the removal of a carious lesion. The chemical adhesion available to both enamel and dentine has been shown to reinforce remaining tooth structure as well as preventing microleakage, and the fluoride release will assist in remineralizing adjacent teeth. Some of the cements are aesthetic and some are radiopaque. They are all moderately easy to place and the only real limitation is that, at present, none of them is strong enough to withstand heavy occlusal stress.

However, they can be regarded as an adequate dentine replacement so that, if the cement can be given sufficient support by sound enamel, there is no need to remove more than the carious lesion. Adhesion to the remaining tooth structure will support the enamel and fluoride release will help to remineralize any demineralized enamel surrounding the lesion. All that is necessary is access to the lesion, with sufficient visibility to ensure removal of all active caries and infected dentine. If, upon completion of the cavity design, it appears that there is too much tooth lost to be able to rely entirely upon glass-ionomer cement, then it should be used as a dentine substitute and the enamel can be replaced with a more substantial material, such as composite resin or amalgam.

This concept has opened up new frontiers in the conservation of natural tooth structure, along with the provision of entirely aesthetic restorations. Any new lesion should be approached in the first instance with the most conservative plan in mind. The initial lesion, prior to complete penetration through the enamel, will almost certainly repair through remineralization. Once the dentine is involved, some degree of surgical intervention becomes necessary and this should also be carried out in the most conservative manner. Using one of

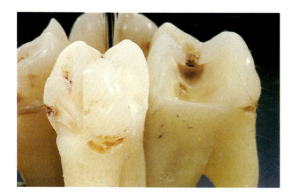

Figure 6.1

An extracted tooth has been sectioned to show three different carious lesions and the direction of penetration of the advancing caries. Note the two stages of the Class I occlusal lesions. On the left the caries has only just penetrated through the fissure and entered the dentine, but on the right the pulp is now involved. The caries has penetrated to a depth that is twice as deep as it is wide and has followed the direction of the dentinal tubules. The proximal lesion on the left has entered the enamel on a narrow front and then progressed inwards and downwards along the path of the dentinal tubules. This pattern of attack is significant in the design of cavities which are intended to remove caries only and minimize the loss of further tooth structure.

the designs discussed in this section, the lesion should be opened up to determine the extent of the problem. If the carious lesion proves to be minimal, it may be restored with the appropriate glass-ionomer cement. If it is a little larger, it may be necessary to cover the cement with composite resin. If the lesion is larger still, other materials, such as amalgam or gold, may have to be utilized.

Suggested cavity design

The following modifications are suggested as being appropriate for restoration with glass-ionomer cement, either alone or in combination, and will be dealt with in turn:

- Class I/fissure seal
- Internal fossa cavities (tunnels)
  Class II proximal
  Class II occlusal
  Class III buccal or lingual
- Combination amalgam and glass-ionomer cement

The first two groups are designed to preserve remaining tooth structure and all new carious lesions should be assessed with these designs in view. If the ultimate cavity proves to be too large, or the occlusal stress too great for restoration in glass-ionomer cement alone, then reinforcement with composite resin or amalgam may be indicated.

The progress of caries into the dentine is illustrated in Figure 6.1. It should be noted that demineralization follows the path of the dentinal tubules and, at least in the early stages, advances on a relatively narrow front. This means a lesion can generally be removed through a very conservative opening in the enamel and its surrounding tooth structure can be maintained. In fact, in the presence of the adhesion available with glass-ionomer cement and composite resin, the intrinsic strength of the crown can be restored very close to the original.

Maintenance of the anatomy of the occlusal surfaces and the subtle curves of the proximal contact areas is very important. These cavity designs offer the possibility of achieving this ideal and deserve careful consideration.

Class I/fissure seal

The conventional G. V. Black design Class I cavity required the removal of all fissures because of the difficulty of finishing an amalgam restoration part way along a fissure. The mechanical broadening of fissures in the enamel, through to and including the dentine, weakens the remaining tooth structure and is therefore undesirable.

Glass-ionomer cements have been shown to be suitable materials for use as a fissure seal, provided that they are properly handled. Also, as long as they are well supported by remaining tooth structure, they can be used to restore small occlusal cavities. Therefore, the combined Class I/fissure seal is a very conservative and desirable alternative to the Class I amalgam.

Cavity design

If there is radiographic evidence of caries, confirming an apparent colour change under the enamel in relation to an occlusal pit or fissure, then the enamel must be removed from this area to disclose the extent of the problem. Good lighting and magnification with loupes is necessary. The lesion should be opened conservatively through the enamel and the caries only removed, without enlarging the access any more than is necessary.

The remaining fissures should be carefully examined for evidence of further carious involvement. As fissures often have constrictions towards the occlusal entrance, this may be difficult to determine (Figure 6.3). If in doubt, a very fine tapered diamond stone at intermediate high speed (40 000 revolutions/min) under air/water spray should be used to open the constriction without completely penetrating the enamel through to the dentine (Figure 6.5). All fissures should be explored as necessary and opened further only if active caries is present (Figure 6.6).

Instruments required (see Box E, page 120)

- Small tapered diamond stone at intermediate high speed (40 000 revolutions/min) under air/water spray, to open the carious lesion
- very fine diamond point, to follow out the fissures
- small round burs, sizes 1/011-016, for caries removal.

Material to use

As it will be necessary later to monitor possible recurrent caries, it is suggested that a radiopaque cement be used.

- Type II.1: Some Type II.1 cements are radiopaque and all have excellent aesthetics. They are slow to achieve water balance and therefore require protection on removal of the matrix with a generous layer of low-viscosity, light-activated resin bond or two layers of varnish. It is also possible to keep such a restoration isolated with a short strip of Stomahesive bandage applied to the tooth and soft tissue immediately on removal of the matrix.
- Type II.2: Fast setting and radiopaque, but aesthetics are not always acceptable. They can be cut back immediately after setting and covered with composite resin to improve aesthetics.
- Type III: If Type III lining cements are to stand on their own with no cover, the powder/liquid ratio must be at least 3:1. If a thinner mix is used or aesthetics is a problem, they must be lightly cut back and covered with composite resin.

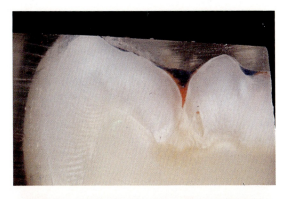

Figure 6.2

Section through the crown of an extracted tooth showing a simple, open-fissure pattern with wide access which has been restored to its full depth with a glass-ionomer cement (dyed red and blue).

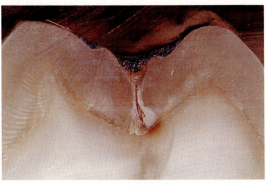

Figure 6.3

Section through an extracted tooth showing the restriction part way down the fissure. This is a common problem which limits the ability of a fissure seal to penetrate to the full depth of a fissure and may lead to failure. Note the demineralization along the walls and at the base of the fissure. Sealing the entry to the fissure will probably arrest this activity but caries in the dentine cannot be assessed without exploration.

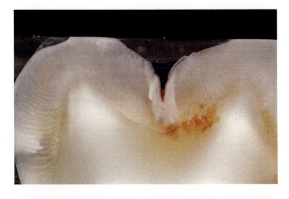

Figure 6.4

Section through the crown of a tooth, showing a relatively open fissure with demineralization on both walls and some dentine involvement. Exploration of this fissure is also justifiable.

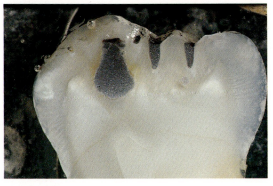

Figure 6.5

A further specimen sectioned mesio-distally following restoration with Ketac Silver (see Figures 6.6–6.10). There are two minor fissures opened very conservatively, with a third opened sufficiently to allow removal of a small area of caries.

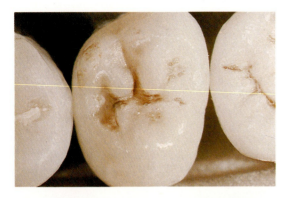

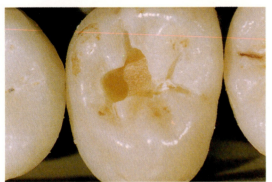

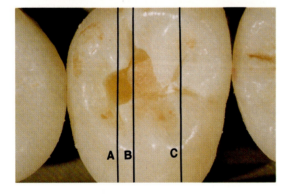

Simulated Class I/fissure seal

Figure 6.6

The occlusal surface of an extracted third molar showing the typical convoluted fissure pattern. The central fossa will catch a fine probe and it is reasonable to expect to find caries beneath. The remaining fissures are difficult to judge and should be explored.

Figure 6.7

a Preparation of the cavity in the tooth shown in Figure 6.6 revealed a moderate amount of caries in the central fossa and minor involvement of the fissures radiating out across the occlusal surface. These were opened very conservatively with a very fine diamond point, without completely penetrating the enamel (see Box E, page 120). Having determined that these fissures were free of caries, the cavity was restored with Ketac Silver.

b The tooth was sectioned three times in a bucco-lingual direction for further examination (Figures 6.8–6.10).

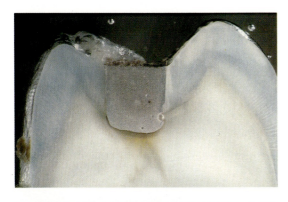

Figure 6.8

Slice A shows the mesial pit which was carious and has been satisfactorily restored with the cement.

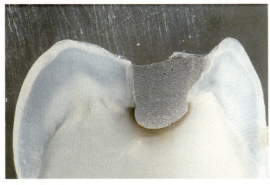

Figure 6.9

Slice B runs along the buccal fissure and shows the way it is ramped up to the occlusal surface without fully penetrating the enamel.

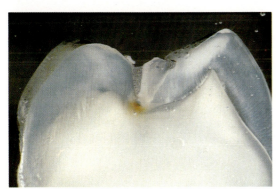

Figure 6.10

Slice C crosses the two distal fissures and confirms that the enamel is again not penetrated and has been satisfactorily sealed with the cement.

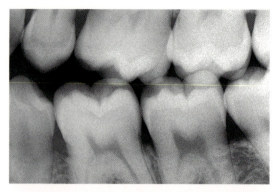

Clinical placement

Class I/fissure seal

Figure 6.11

Bitewing radiograph of the patient's left-hand side, showing a probable carious lesion under the central fissure of the lower-first molar.

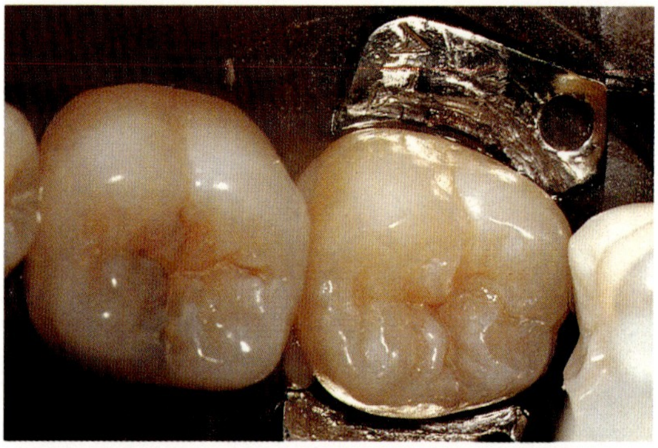

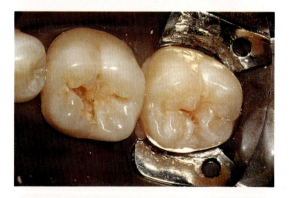

Figure 6.12

An occlusal view of the lower-left first and second molars. Note the subtle colour change in the central fissure of the first molar confirming the radiographic view. The fissures in the second molar are also deep enough to warrant fissure sealing.

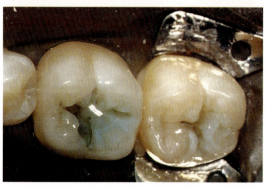

Figure 6.13

The cavity has been prepared very conservatively in the first molar with the caries removed and the remaining fissure opened very narrowly. The fissures in the second molar have been widened a little with the tip of a very fine diamond bur, just to remove the constriction, but the enamel has not been totally penetrated (see Box E, page 120).

Figure 6.14

Immediately cavity preparation is complete, the teeth are conditioned with 10 per cent poly(acrylic acid) for 15 seconds, then washed thoroughly and dried lightly but not dehydrated.

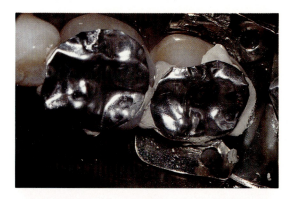

Figure 6.15

Lead-foil matrices have been prepared, using the foil from the back of a standard dental radiograph (see Box F, page 121). A section large enough to cover the occlusal of the tooth has been cut out and then a layer of low-viscosity, light-activated resin bonding agent has been painted on the undersurface and light activated. The cavities have been restored with Ketac Silver and the matrices positioned.

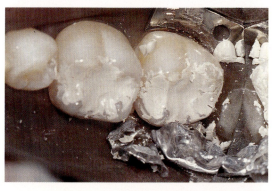

Figure 6.16

At approximately 4 minutes from the start of mix, the excess cement is tested for degree of set and the matrices peeled off.

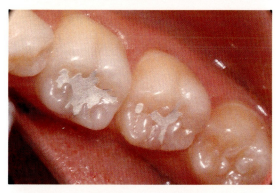

Figure 6.17

Because Ketac Silver is a fast-setting material, it can now be trimmed immediately under air/water spray, using very fine diamonds followed by graded rubber abrasive points.

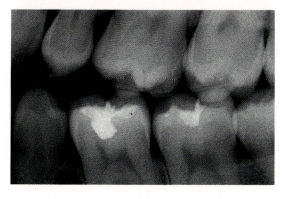

Figure 6.18

Bitewing radiograph of the restorations. Further progress of active caries can be monitored radiographically as required.

Internal fossa cavities (tunnels)

The physical properties of glass-ionomer cements are such that, if they are to be used on the occlusal surface of a tooth, they require support from surrounding tooth structure. Although occlusal load varies from one patient to another, building an entire occlusal surface, including the marginal ridge, with glass-ionomer cement is generally contraindicated. This has led to the development of an extremely conservative approach to the proximal carious lesion, where microsurgical techniques are aimed at removal of the caries without involving any more sound tooth structure than is necessary.

Glass-ionomer cements are the material of choice for this technique because they are relatively easy to place in small cavities, and the adhesion to remaining tooth structure gives a degree of support to the undermined marginal ridge sufficient to prevent its subsequent breakdown. In addition, the fluoride leaching from the cement will assist in remineralizing the surrounding enamel to the extent that it is not necessary to remove all demineralized enamel.

The cavities prepared on these principles have been variously described as internal occlusal fossa cavities or tunnels, and their design requires excellent lighting and vision, including the use of magnification with loupes. All new Class II carious lesions should be viewed as possible candidates for this cavity design because if, having begun this procedure, the marginal ridge fails, then a conventional Class II design can be developed without unnecessary loss of sound tooth structure.

The following classification of 'tunnel cavities' is suggested:

- Class II proximal: the proximal surface of the tooth adjacent to the lesion has already been opened in a conventional Class II cavity design, thereby allowing access for a direct approach to the lesion to be treated (Figures 6.19–6.24).
- Class II occlusal: the marginal ridge is still intact and the proximal carious lesion is relatively limited in its penetration into dentine. The adjacent tooth is sound, so access is obtained through the occlusal surface (Figures 6.29–6.35).
- Class III buccal or lingual: generally there has been some degree of gingival recession and often there is an existing Class II restoration or a crown. Further carious attack has taken place on the root surface and, depending on problems of access, the approach will be from the buccal or the lingual (Figures 6.47–6.52).

Class II proximal

Cavity design

Following the preparation of a conventional Class II cavity in the adjacent tooth, the full extent of the demineralized area of the lesion to be treated will be visible. The depth of penetration of the carious dentine can be assessed from the radiograph, but will not be fully realized until access is gained through the enamel. The angle of approach with a bur will be dictated largely by the adjacent tooth, and this may make it difficult to clean up under the marginal ridge. As the caries will generally progress inwards and downwards along the course of the dentinal tubules, this limitation is generally not a problem (Figure 6.1). All of the demineralized enamel and the carious dentine can be removed in a conventional manner but the strength of the marginal ridge must be maintained as far as possible (Figures 6.19–6.24).

Instruments required (see Box E, page 120)

- A small tapered diamond stone at intermediate high speed (40 000 revolutions/min) under air/water spray to open the enamel lesion
- small round burs, sizes 1/011–016, for caries removal
- access for hand instruments is limited, but the MCL double-bladed chisel may be useful.

Materials for restoration

As the restoration will be hidden by the adjacent tooth, it is necessary to use a cement that is radiopaque. The Type II.2 restorative reinforced cement is the material of choice because it is fast setting and can be polished immediately after placement, and before placement of the adjacent restoration. It has the additional advantage of a higher abrasion resistance and will therefore withstand regular cleaning with dental floss without undue wear.

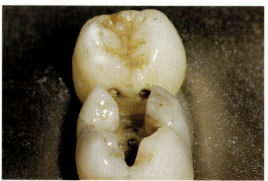

Simulated Class II Proximal

Figure 6.19

Restoration of a lesion in an extracted tooth. A large cavity has been opened in the mesial of a first molar, revealing a proximal lesion in the distal of the second bicuspid.

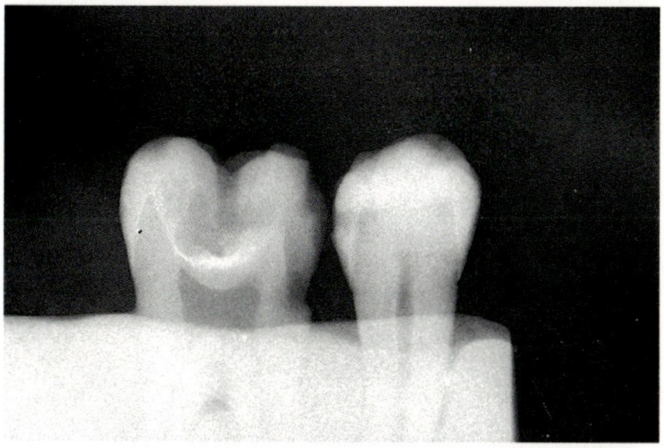

Figure 6.20

A radiograph confirms the extent of the lesion.

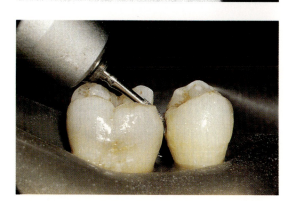

Figure 6.21

The presence of the adjacent tooth limits the angle at which the bur can be manipulated in the handpiece. However, as the caries will penetrate down the dentinal tubules away from the occlusal, this angle of approach generally coincides with the progress of the lesion (Figure 6.1). The full extent of the enamel lesion can be removed and the carious dentine can be dealt with (see Box E, page 120).

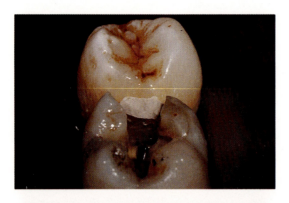

Figure 6.22

The cavity can now be conditioned and restored with Ketac Silver. Five minutes from the start of mix, the cement can be contoured and polished completely.

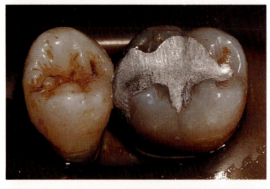

Figure 6.23

A matrix can now be placed on the adjacent molar and the restoration of choice carried out.

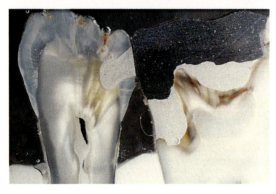

Figure 6.24

The assembled teeth have been sectioned mesio-distally to show the design of the tunnel cavity. Note that the design of the cavity follows the dentinal tubules and that this coincides with the direction of penetration of the caries (Figure 6.1).

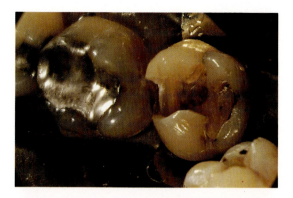

Clinical placement

Class II proximal

Figure 6.25

On opening the mesial cavity in an upper-right second molar, a lesion became obvious in the distal of the first molar. Radiographically, there was very little penetration into the dentine and so a proximal approach was carried out.

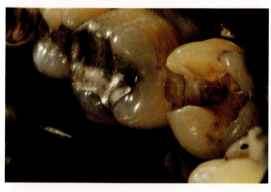

Figure 6.26

The completed cavity showing that the enamel wall is caries free.

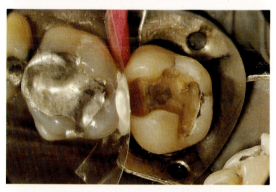

Figure 6.27

A short length of mylar strip is used as a matrix and, after conditioning the cavity, this is wedged into place and the cement is syringed and tamped into the cavity.

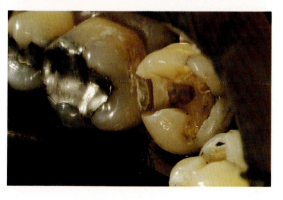

Figure 6.28

The matrix can be removed at 4 minutes from the start of mix and the cement trimmed and polished immediately.

Class II occlusal

The demineralized enamel in a Class II carious lesion is generally an elliptical area immediately below the contact area between adjacent teeth. There will often be an intact marginal ridge with a reasonably strong wall of enamel occlusal to the lesion. If this can be maintained, the adhesion to the glass-ionomer cement will reinforce it and the failure rate is low.

The dentine lesion may be more extensive than assessed on the radiograph and it will generally penetrate inwards and downwards along the path of the dentinal tubules. There must be full visual access to the caries if it is to be removed completely. Good lighting and magnification using loupes is necessary.

Cavity design

The direction of progress of the early carious lesion on the proximal surface immediately below the proximal contact area should be noted (Figure 6.1). The initial approach to the carious dentine will be through the occlusal enamel just medial to the marginal ridge. There is generally a pit or an extension of a fissure in this region which will be the logical starting point. Entry should be made through this area, with the bur angled mesially or distally aiming for the carious dentine (Figure 6.31). The lesion may then be located visually. To open the access cavity and improve visibility the cavity is re-entered, keeping the tip of the bur in approximately the same position. The bur may then be uprighted towards the marginal ridge and leaned buccally and lingually (Figure 6.32). This will develop a somewhat triangular entry to a funnel-shaped approach, allowing complete access to the caries (Figure 6.33). The caries should be removed and the extent of the problem determined. The gingival margin of the enamel lesion will now be visible, but the occlusal margin remains difficult to visualize and assess. In view of the remineralizing potential of the glass-ionomer cements, it is acceptable to leave some demineralized enamel, provided that the demineralization is confined to the outer half of the enamel only (Figure 6.35).

Instruments required (see Box E, page 120)

- Small, tapered diamond stone at intermediate high speed (40 000 revolutions/min) with air/water spray, to open the occlusal enamel
- small round burs, sizes 1/011–016, for caries removal
- long, fine-shank bur for difficult access
- access for hand instruments is limited, but the MCL double-bladed chisel may be useful.

Materials for restoration

Because monitoring for recurrent caries is necessary, a radiopaque cement is mandatory. In areas where aesthetics is important a Type II.1 restorative aesthetic cement is acceptable, provided that it is radiopaque. Otherwise, the Type II.2 is the material of choice. It is fast setting and its high abrasion resistance is an advantage. If aesthetics is important, the occlusal should be covered with composite resin, using the sandwich technique.

Before beginning cavity preparation, a metal matrix strip should be placed interproximally, both to protect the adjacent tooth during cavity preparation and also to prevent the cement from sticking to it during placement (see Box F, page 121). The matrix must be wedged firmly into place (see Box G, page 122). On completing the cavity it should be conditioned with 10 per cent poly(acrylic acid) for 15 seconds, then the cement tamped into place in at least two increments, using a small plastic sponge (see Figure 7.25) to minimize porosity and to ensure that excess cement escapes through the enamel lesion. Proper adaptation of the cement to the proximal enamel margins is probably the most difficult aspect of this restoration. Application of a further soft metal matrix to the occlusal surface will ensure complete placement of the cement under positive pressure.

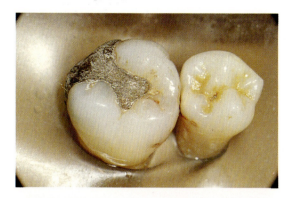

Simulated Class II occlusal

Figure 6.29

A simulated model for the preparation of a Class II occlusal approach internal fossa cavity. There is a cavity on the proximal surface of the molar tooth and it will be approached through the mesial pit on the occlusal.

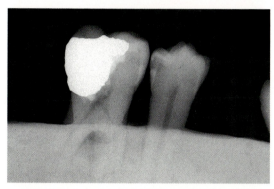

Figure 6.30

A radiograph of the two teeth showing the extent of the cavity. The cavity on the distal of the bicuspid is not suitable for a tunnel approach because the lesion is too close to the marginal ridge and it is likely to collapse during cavity preparation. A so-called marginal ridge approach is recommended under these circumstances (see Figures 4.2 and 4.3).

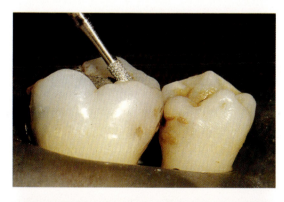

Figure 6.31

The initial approach is through the mesial pit with the bur aimed at the carious lesion, until the lesion is reached.

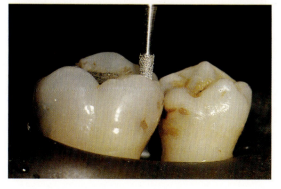

Figure 6.32

The bur is uprighted, keeping the tip in the same place, and leaning the bur to the buccal and the lingual to produce a funnel-type access to the lesion. The strength of the marginal ridge must be maintained.

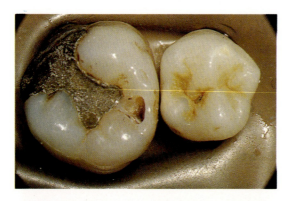

Figure 6.33

The caries is removed using small, round burs. If access permits, the enamel lesion may be cleaned with the MCL double-bladed chisel. Note the triangular outline of the occlusal entry cavity.

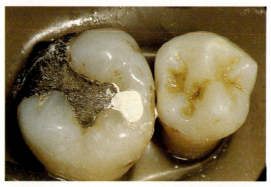

Figure 6.34

The restored cavity, which shows again the triangular outline and the minimal tooth loss required to restore the lesion.

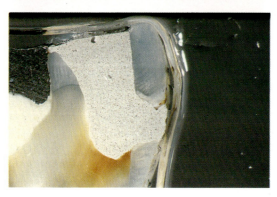

Figure 6.35

A cross-section of the same restoration. Note the substantial band of sound enamel under the marginal ridge and the sound placement of the cement with minimum porosity and voids. There is good adaptation of the cement to the gingival margin of the enamel lesion, but the occlusal margin is the problem area. However, because of the potential for remineralization, there is some degree of latitude.

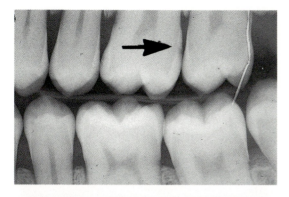

Clinical placement

Class II occlusal tunnel

Figure 6.36

A radiograph reveals a small carious lesion at the distal of the upper-right first molar.

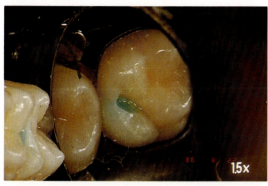

Figure 6.37

The access cavity on the occlusal is approximately triangular in outline, maintaining the strength of the marginal ridge. The caries is cleaned out with a small, round bur and then the cavity conditioned with 10 per cent poly(acrylic acid) for 10 seconds.

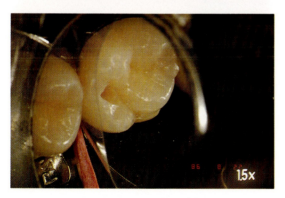

Figure 6.38

A matrix is wedged firmly into place using a short length of mylar strip.

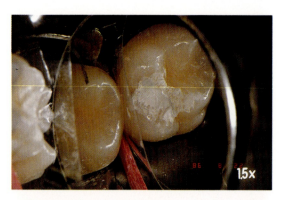

Figure 6.39

The cement is placed in at least two increments, and tamped into place with a small plastic sponge. A small soft-metal matrix is placed over the occlusal to force the cement into place and left until it has set.

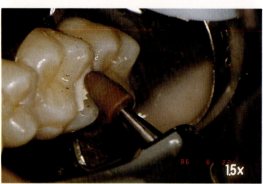

Figure 6.40

At 5 minutes from the start of mix, the excess is trimmed and the cement polished with mild abrasive cups and points under air/water spray.

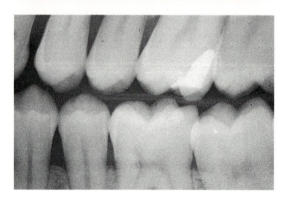

Figure 6.41

Radiograph of the completed restoration. If aesthetics is of concern, the occlusal 2 mm can be trimmed back and composite resin applied using the sandwich technique.

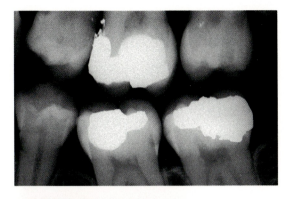

Class II tunnel through an existing cavity

Figure 6.42

Bitewing radiograph reveals a small carious lesion at the distal of the lower-left first molar. The existing occlusal Class I amalgam is classified as requiring replacement, so the distal lesion will be approached through the amalgam cavity.

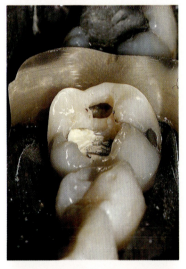

Figure 6.43

The amalgam has been removed and the carious lesion identified and cleaned out. Access under these circumstances is straightforward and visibility is not a problem. The metal matrix was placed early to avoid damage to the adjacent tooth during cavity preparation.

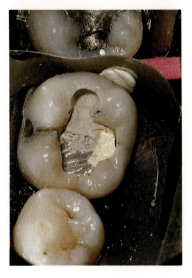

Figure 6.44

Ketac Silver has been syringed into the cavity and tamped into place with a small plastic sponge. Note the excess cement that has extruded out beyond the matrix, thus ensuring good adaptation to the enamel. The same cement has been spread out on the floor of the cavity as a lining.

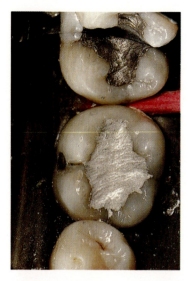

Figure 6.45

Amalgam has now been replaced in the main cavity as it was considered too large to be restored in glass-ionomer cement alone.

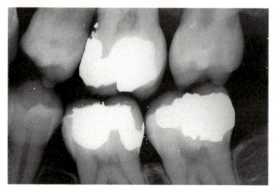

Figure 6.46

Radiograph showing the completed restoration.

Class III buccal or lingual

Patients who have suffered bone loss and migration of the epithelial attachment may demonstrate carious lesions on the root surface well beyond the normal contact area. These lesions can arise in relation to existing restorations as root-surface caries, or be the result of functionally opening contacts and resultant food impaction. There will be a considerable amount of sound tooth structure or an otherwise acceptable restoration occlusal to the lesion. The conservative approach is to enter the lesion from either the buccal or the lingual, whichever provides the easier access and visibility, and remove only the caries, with minimal destruction of remaining tooth structure or restoration. The available ionic bond, fluoride release and high tissue tolerance make glass-ionomer cement the material of choice to restore these cavities (see Figure 6.52).

Cavity design

Access to the cavity will generally be available from either the buccal or the lingual. Entry is made with a small, tapered diamond stone and the access enlarged both occlusally and gingivally to determine the extent of the problem. Sufficient of the existing restoration must be removed to expose any caries that may have progressed occlusally. During removal of the caries it is preferable to try to maintain a flat wall on the side opposite to the entry cavity (Figure 6.50). This facilitates construction of a matrix and placement of the ultimate restoration. A small amount of positive retention in the occlusal and the gingival walls should always be developed. In view of the lack of microleakage with glass-ionomer cements, it is possible to leave a small amount of softened dentine on the axial wall if a pulp exposure is otherwise likely.

Instruments required (see Box E, page 120)

- Small, tapered diamond stone at intermediate high speed (40 000 revolutions/min) with air/water spray, to open into the lesion at the expense of both tooth structure and old restoration
- small round burs, sizes 1/011–016, for caries removal
- long shank round burs may be required for deep access
- round bur size 1/011, for retention
- access for hand instruments is limited.

Materials for restoration

These cavities often pose problems of access and may even be sub-gingival. They also need to be monitored for possible recurrent caries. Therefore the Type II.2 restorative reinforced cement is the material of choice. There is unlikely to be a problem with aesthetics.

A matrix can be constructed from either a mylar strip or a metal band (see Box F, page 121). The metal band should be lightly vaselined to prevent it sticking to the cement and wedged firmly in place. If a wooden wedge is likely to distort the matrix, a pledget of cotton soaked in a light-activated resin bonding agent may be used. This is placed gently where required and the resin light activated (see Box G, page 122). This will provide sufficient support to prevent distortion during placement.

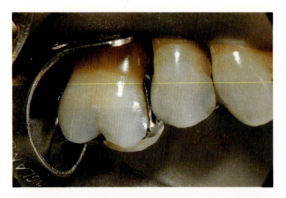

Clinical placement

Class III buccal tunnel

Figure 6.47

An upper-right first molar has over-erupted and now shows root-surface caries beyond the gingival margin of an old amalgam. The amalgam is considered to be otherwise satisfactory, so a buccal approach to the carious lesion is the method of choice.

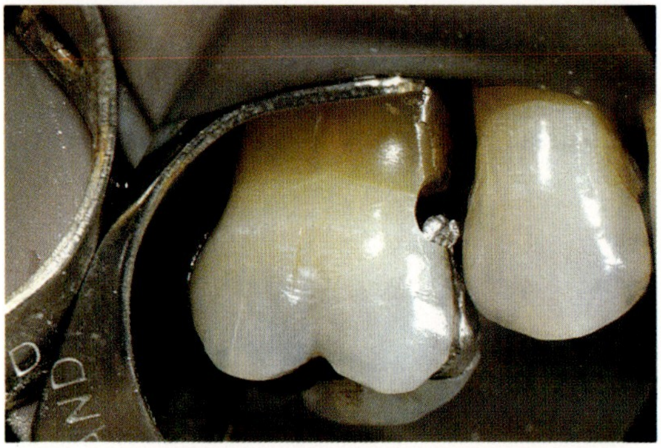

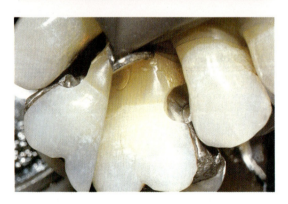

Figure 6.48

The initial approach is at the expense of enamel and dentine only to determine the extent of the problem.

Figure 6.49

Having determined the extent of the problem, the cavity outline is completed, including the removal of some of the old amalgam to gain full access.

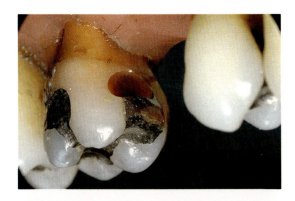

Figure 6.50

A simulated cavity on a similar extracted tooth to demonstrate the extent of the cavity design. Retention has been provided with shallow grooves in the occlusal and gingival walls, and the lingual wall has been retained as far as possible to act as a base against which to place the cement.

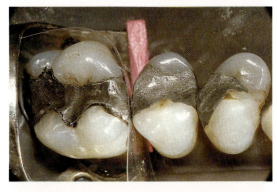

Figure 6.51

A short length of mylar strip is wedged into place as a matrix, and the cavity is conditioned, washed and dried.

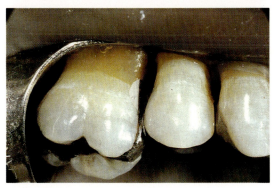

Figure 6.52

The cement is tamped into place in at least two increments, and at 6 minutes from the start of mix it can be trimmed and polished.

Combination amalgam and glass-ionomer cement

Teeth that are extensively broken down as a result of repeated caries attacks followed by multiple restorations can pose a problem if a new amalgam restoration is to be constructed. Similar problems arise following root-surface caries beyond an existing restoration where a Class III tunnel approach is not possible. Access is not always available to all areas of the cavity at the same time and construction of a matrix may be complex. One alternative in these cases may be the restoration of one section of the cavity with a fast-setting glass-ionomer cement to act as a foundation and to overcome the problem of multiple access angles. The cement may not be strong enough to withstand the occlusal stress on its own, but overlaid with a substantial bulk of amalgam the load is sufficiently distributed for the result to be satisfactory (Figures 6.61–6.63).

Cavity design

All old restorative material must be removed and visibility and access gained to the entire lesion. In the area to be restored with the cement, it is only necessary to ensure that the walls are caries free. If there is any doubt about retention, minimum grooves may be provided in appropriate regions. If there is less than 0.5 mm of remaining dentine over the pulp, a small quantity of a quick-setting calcium hydroxide may be placed where required. The cavity can then be conditioned with 10 per cent poly(acrylic acid) overfilled with glass-ionomer cement and allowed to set. The cement may then be cut back to produce a satisfactory design for the amalgam. Some degree of chemical union can be developed between glass-ionomer cement and amalgam by applying a light coat of 45 per cent poly(acrylic acid) to the newly set glass-ionomer cement and leaving it in place for 1 minute. The excess acid should be gently dried off, but not washed off. The amalgam can then be condensed onto the cement with the development of chemical union between the two. A small amount of mechanical interlock should also be provided to ensure stability in the amalgam.

Instruments required (see Box E, page 120)

- Ultra-high speed (250 000 revolutions/min and above) with diamonds and tungsten carbide burs as required to outline the basic cavity
- small, tapered diamond stone at intermediate high speed (40 000 revolutions/min) under air/water spray, to refine the outline
- round burs, sizes 1/011–016, for caries removal
- tapered fissure burs, for retentive grooves
- self-threading pins, to enhance retention
- hand instruments, to refine the margins.

Materials for restoration

A fast-setting cement is required to allow completion of the amalgam at the same appointment. It is essential also that the material be radiopaque so that it can be monitored radiographically for recurrent caries. The Type II.2 cermet cement is thus the material of choice.

A short length of either mylar strip or a metal matrix band may serve as a matrix (see Box F, page 121), supported with a wooden wedge or a small pledget of cotton soaked in a light-activated resin bond, positioned and light activated (see Box G, page 122). The cement is then introduced and tamped into place using a small plastic sponge (Figure 7.25) to adapt it to the cavity walls and to minimize porosity. The same cement can be spread over the pulpal floor and axial wall as a lining (Figure 6.56). An excess of cement should always be placed and then cut back to refine the amalgam cavity design. Five minutes from the start of mix, the cement can be cut back under air/water spray at intermediate high speed, a conventional metal matrix can be placed and wedged and the amalgam can be packed immediately.

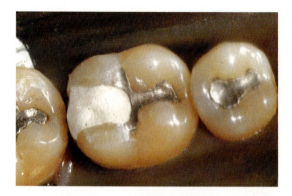

Clinical placement

Class II Ketac Silver/amalgam restoration

Figure 6.53

A large Ketac Silver restoration of a distal Class II lesion in the lower-right first molar. There is an open contact with the adjacent tooth because of the difficulty of contouring a restoration of this size in Ketac Silver.

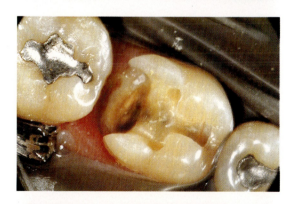

Figure 6.54

Bitewing radiograph shows that the Ketac Silver has been poorly placed at the gingival, that there is a rough proximal contour and that caries is still present. Note recurrent caries in the opposing first and second molars and a distal cavity in the lower-right second bicuspid.

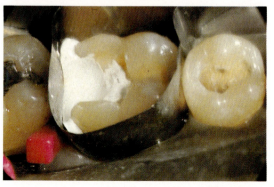

Figure 6.55

Cavity design has been completed in the lower first molar. The rubber dam has been lifted mesially to show the condition of the gingival tissue in relation to the gingival margin of the cavity. The tissue tolerance of the original Ketac Silver was such that the gingival tissue remained moderately healthy.

Figure 6.56

A standard metal matrix has been placed without a matrix retainer and gently wedged at the gingival to give a degree of support without distortion (see Box G, page 122). The cavity was conditioned with 10 per cent poly(acrylic acid) for 10 seconds and then overfilled with Ketac Silver which was tamped into place with a small plastic sponge (see Figure 7.25). It was left to set 6 minutes.

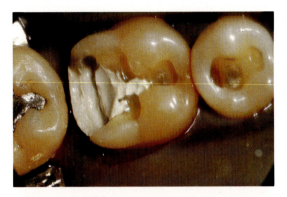

Figure 6.57

The cement was contoured under air/water spray at intermediate high speed to just below the contact area with the adjacent second molar. Normal mechanical interlocks cut in the remaining tooth structure support the amalgam and a groove cut in the Ketac Silver ensures the interlock. A thin layer of Ketac Silver has been left on the pulpal floor as a normal lining. A very small quantity of 45 per cent poly(acrylic acid) can now be applied on a cotton pledget to the Ketac Silver and left for 1 minute. Any excess should be wiped off but not washed off.

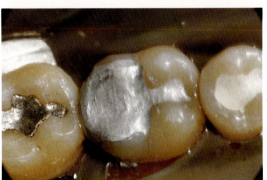

Figure 6.58

A normal amalgam matrix can now be applied and the amalgam condensed as usual. Note the protective cavity design. The tunnel cavity in the second bicuspid has been restored with Ketac Silver also. The occlusal of this restoration was subsequently replaced with composite resin.

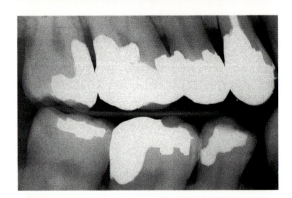

Figure 6.59

Bitewing radiograph showing the finished restoration in the first molar as well as the tunnel restoration in the second bicuspid. The upper right first and second molars have also been restored with amalgam over Ketac Silver in a similar fashion.

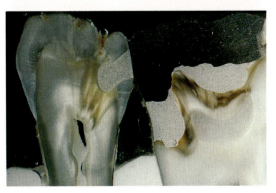

Figure 6.60

A simulated restoration on an extracted tooth sectioned mesio-distally to show the cement occupying the gingival half of the cavity and spread over the pulpal floor as well as a lining. Note that there has been a small amount of mechanical retention provided along the gingival floor to compensate for the relative weakness of the ionic bond between dentine and Ketac Silver.

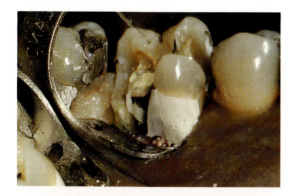

Class II amalgam/Class V Ketac Silver

Figure 6.61

An extensive cavity in a lower-right first molar involving mesial, distal, occlusal and buccal surfaces. Because of the difficulty of packing the buccal extension with amalgam at the same time as the rest of the cavity, the buccal was restored first with Ketac Silver.

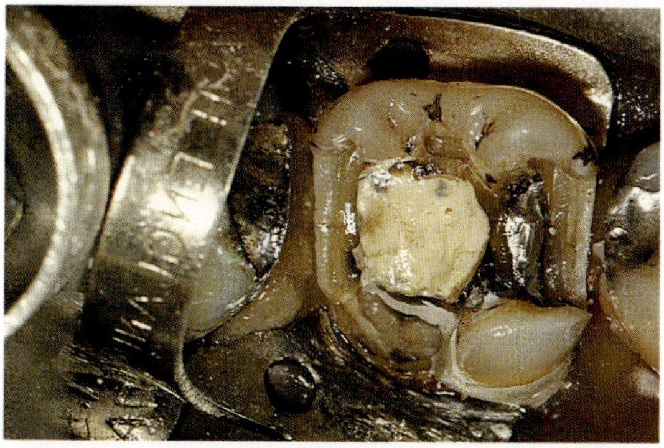

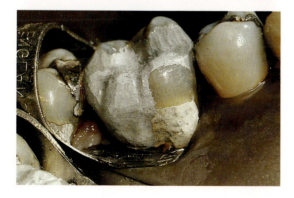

Figure 6.62

At 6 minutes from the start of mix, the cement was trimmed back and the final cavity designed for amalgam.

Figure 6.63

The amalgam has been placed and the restoration is complete.

7 Instructions for dental assistants

As with all dental materials, the dental assistant plays an important part in correct handling and clinical success. This section is therefore designed to help the dental assistant to understand the handling requirements of the glass-ionomer cements. As all three types are essentially the same from a chemical point of view, they can all be discussed under the same headings. There is nothing particularly difficult in the storage, dispensing or mixing of these cements. Precision and understanding are a necessary part of good dental assisting, and the following points should always be observed when handling the glass-ionomer cements.

Storage of cement in bottles

Powders or liquids supplied by different manufacturers or of different types must **never** be interchanged. They are all different and an interchange of components will destroy properties.

Because the glass-ionomer cements are water-based cements, they will always be subject to further loss or uptake of water. Therefore both powder and liquid bottles should remain firmly closed at all times (Figure 7.1).

With some of the materials available, the liquid supplied is a type of poly(alkenoic acid). With others, the poly(alkenoic acid) has been dehydrated and is already incorporated in the powder. In this case, the liquid will be water or a solution of tartaric acid.

If the liquid being used is poly(alkenoic acid), it will be subject to water uptake and the bottle should remain firmly closed. In addition, it will tend to age and thicken over a period of time. Within 12 months of manufacture, the viscosity may increase to the stage where it flows very slowly and is difficult to dispense accurately. The liquid can be thinned down as follows:

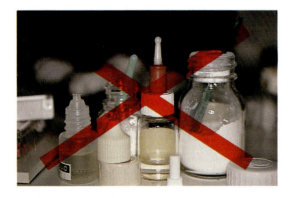

Figure 7.1

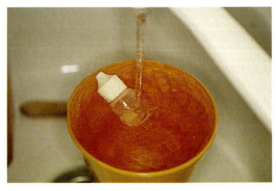

Figure 7.2

- Immerse the entire bottle, with the lid on, in water at 75 °C (167 °F) for 15 minutes. Stand the bottle in a rubber bowl and let the water from the hot tap run over it. The bottle will float on the top of the water but the temperature will be about right (Figure 7.2).
- Test it at 15 minutes and see that the viscosity has come back to normal.
- Let it cool off again before using it.

The liquids should **never** be stored in the refrigerator, but storage of the powder and the mixing slab in the refrigerator will marginally lengthen working time (Figure 7.3). The difference will not be great, but, where the office is not air-conditioned, or the average temperature is high, it is worth while because it will take the pressure off the clinical handling.

- Make sure that the slab is not below the dew point before dispensing the powder.
- Wipe it quite dry with a tissue or there will be a small addition of water to the powder.

Hand dispensing of powder and liquid

If the capsulated varieties of cement are not available, then hand dispensing must be carried out with great care.

- Read the manufacturer's instructions, which will generally suggest that the powder be fluffed up in the bottle first and a level spoonful extracted and dispensed on to the slab.
- Make sure that the spoon is full and that there is no excess powder on the back of the spoon or along the handle.
- Scrape the top of the spoon over the lip on the bottle and be prepared to repeat the measure if there are obvious spaces in the powder (Figure 7.4).

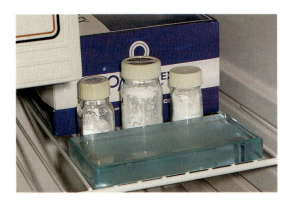

Figure 7.3

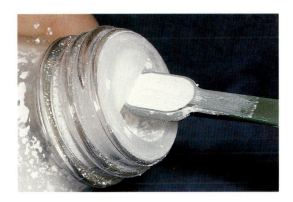

Figure 7.4

If the liquid is poly(acrylic acid), it is difficult to dispense without including an air bubble in the drop, particularly as it becomes more viscous. Dispense in two distinct moves:

- Tip the bottle onto its side first and allow the liquid to run into the spout
- Invert completely before dispensing a drop (Figures 7.5, 7.6). Generally, there will now be a clean drop dispensed with no air bubble included.

If the liquid is water or dilute tartaric acid, care must be taken to dispense only one drop at a time.

- Apply gentle pressure to the rubber cuff at the neck of the bottle, as a vigorous squeeze may produce a squirt rather than a drop (Figure 7.7).

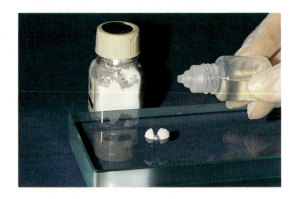

Figure 7.5

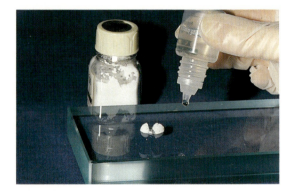

Figure 7.6

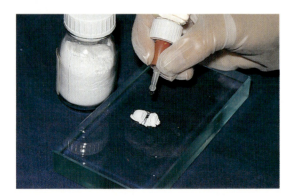

Figure 7.7

Mixing by hand

Most of the manufacturers provide a paper pad on which to mix the cement. This is quite satisfactory provided that the liquid is not left standing on the pad for longer than one minute, because water is likely to soak into the pad from the liquid and alter the powder/liquid ratio. Use of a glass slab is to be recommended because it will not affect the water balance, it can be chilled in the refrigerator and working time can thus be slightly extended (Figure 7.8).

The principle of mixing is simply to fold the powder into the liquid in the shortest possible time (Figures 7.9–7.11).

● Do not spread the mix around the slab and do not spatulate heavily. The object is to wet the surface of each particle of glass powder to develop the matrix, and not to dissolve the entire particles in the liquid. This means that either a steel or a plastic spatula can be used as long as it is handled correctly.

● Divide the powder into two parts. Fold in the first half within 10–15 seconds then add the second half and incorporate it entirely within the next 15 seconds. Keep the mixing to a small area of the slab only and do not continue to spatulate once the powder is all incorporated.

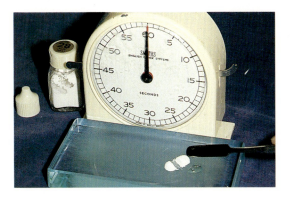

Figure 7.9

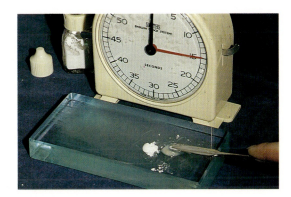

Figure 7.10

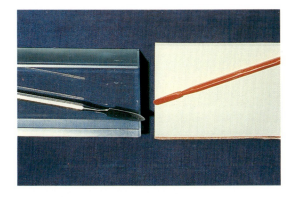

Figure 7.8

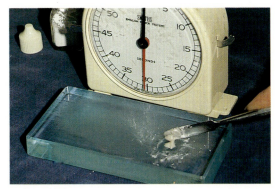

Figure 7.11

Mixing of capsules

In those cements dispensed in capsules, the liquid component is generally a poly(alkeonic acid). This means that care must be taken in collapsing the capsule to see that all the acid has been squeezed out of its sachet.

● If the capsule is activated in a press, apply adequate pressure to the capsule and maintain that pressure for 3 or 4 seconds before releasing and placing the capsule in the machine for mixing (Figure 7.12).

● If the capsule is activated by rotating one half against the other, use adequate force to collapse it (Figure 7.13).

● Note the prescribed mixing time and do not vary it. Use an ultra-high-speed mixing machine, which means one capable of at least 4000 cycles/min. Machines capable of 3000 cycles/min are really not suitable for mixing these cements. It is important to realize that there is considerable variation between different types of machine, and even some variation within machines of the same make. This means that results are not necessarily standard.

● Learn to recognize the time for 'loss of gloss' from the cement mixed by your machine, because placement of the cement after that time will result in loss of adhesion and reduction of physical properties in the final restoration. To test the machine, make a trial mix and time it from the beginning of mix. Express the mix into a pile on a glass slab and watch it carefully. Although difficult to define, there is a point at which the gloss will have gone entirely from the surface. Normally this point should be reached at about 2 minutes from the start of mix.

The time for mixing usually recommended is 10 seconds in a machine capable of 4000 cycles/min. Extension beyond this time up to 15 seconds will reduce working time significantly and is clinically undesirable. Reduction of mixing time to 7 seconds may extend working time to about 2.5 minutes, but there is a risk of having unreacted liquid still present (see Box A, page 6).

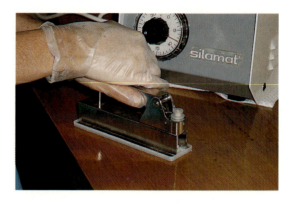

Figure 7.12

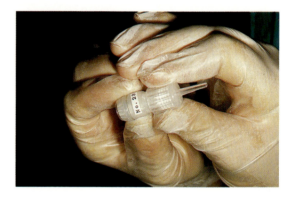

Figure 7.13

- Immediately the capsule is removed from the machine the spout can be bent in the fingers through about 45 degrees for ease of placement of the cement into difficult corners (Figure 7.14).
- Deliver the capsule promptly to the operator. Working time is not long, because of the small temperature rise caused by the high energy of the machine-mixing.

Correct consistency for hand-mixed cements

Type I luting cement

Type I luting cement will be mixed at a powder/liquid ratio of about 1.5:1 and will therefore string up approximately 3–4 cm from the slab (Figures 7.15, 7.16).

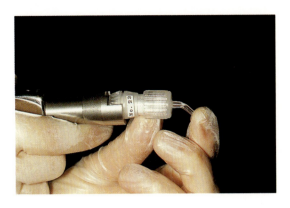

Figure 7.14

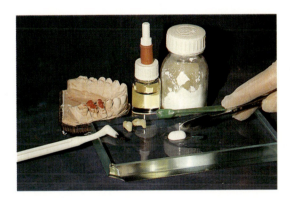

Figure 7.15

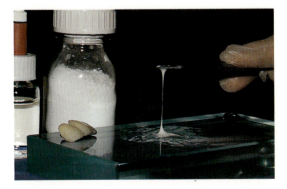

Figure 7.16

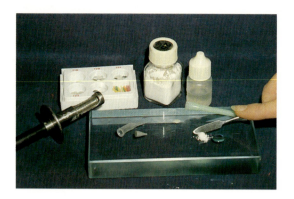

Figure 7.17

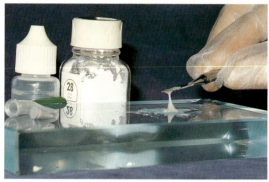

Figure 7.18

Type II.1 restorative aesthetic cements

Type II.1 restorative aesthetic cements will string only 1 cm off the slab but must retain a glossy surface (Figures 7.17, 7.18).

Type II.2 restorative reinforced cements

Type II.2 restorative reinforced cements will have the same powder/liquid ratio as the Type II.1 restorative aesthetic cement. Therefore they will string up approximately 1 cm off the slab and must retain a glossy surface. Working time for the hand-mixed variety will be very short (as these cements are generally capsulated, no illustration is shown).

Type III lining cement

For **lining** amalgams, the powder/liquid ratio will be only 1.5–1.0 so the cement will string up 4–5 cm off the slab (see Figure 7.16).

For **basing out** composite resins, the powder/liquid ratio will be 3:1 or greater, so capsulation is recommended. If hand-mixed, it will string out only 2 cm but must retain a glossy surface (see Figures 7.19, 7.20). Working time will be very short.

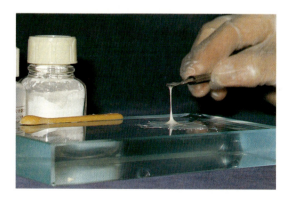

Figure 7.19

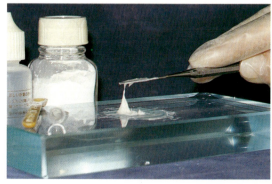

Figure 7.20

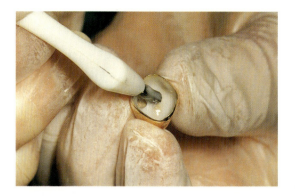

Figure 7.21

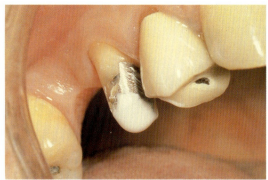

Figure 7.22

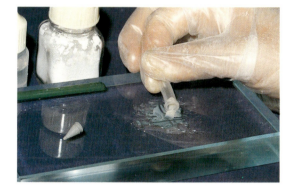

Figure 7.23

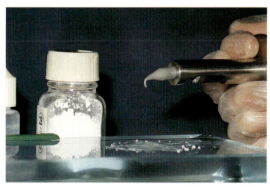

Figure 7.24

Methods of placement

Type I luting cements

Apply with a short, stiff-bristled brush to both the restoration and the tooth (Figures 7.21, 7.22).

Type II.1 restorative aesthetic

Apply for preference in a syringe, for positive placement and reduction of porosity. If hand-mixed, transfer into a Centrix-type disposable syringe (Figures 7.23, 7.24).

Type II.2 restorative reinforced

Apply in a syringe and tamp into place using a small plastic sponge (Figure 7.25). If hand-mixed, transfer into a Centrix-type disposable syringe.

Type III lining cements

Lining amalgam

Apply with calcium hydroxide applicator and flow into place (see Figure 5.8).

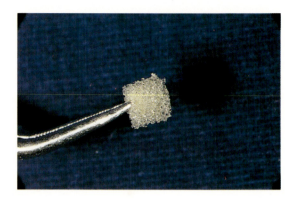

Figure 7.25

For basing

Apply with a syringe and tamp into place with a small plastic sponge (Figure 7.25).

Clean-up procedures

- As soon as the cement has been used, and prior to its setting, completely immerse the slab and the spatula in water. It will then clean off quite readily. The longer it is allowed to set, the more difficult it will be to remove (Figures 7.26–7.27).
- If the cement has inadvertently been allowed to set on the slab or the instruments, then there is no alternative other than to chip it off. Stand it in water for a while first and this will make it easier, but it will still be hard work.

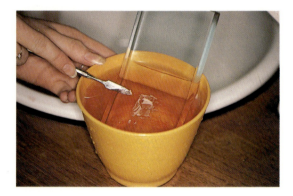

Figure 7.26

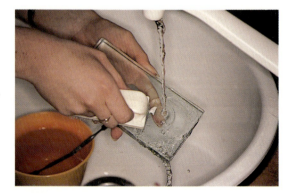

Figure 7.27

8 Condensed instructions: all types

The following instructions are meant to be a brief resumé aimed primarily at the chairside dental assistant. They can be used in place of the printed instructions from manufacturers which often are a little vague and on many occasions are clouded by the use of adjectives extolling the virtues of their particular product.

These instructions can be used as a ready reference for each of the types of material and are brief enough to be kept in the operating room for ready reference by the assistant.

Type I: Luting cements

Dispensing

The powder/liquid ratio is important.
When dispensing the powder, follow the manufacturer's directions. In particular:
- Shake the bottle
- Spoon out the powder carefully.

It is very easy to:
- Have voids in the powder and therefore underdispense
- Have spare powder on the back of the spoon or the handle, and therefore overdispense
When dispensing the liquid:
- Hold the bottle vertically upside-down
- Count the drops.
- Mix half the powder at a time and complete the mix quickly. the chemical reaction begins **immediately**, and prolonged mixing will only break up the newly formed polymer chains.

Conditioning the tooth

Vital tooth

Having removed the temporary restoration and any remaining cement, just wash the tooth with air/water spray and lightly dry it. Do not dehydrate.

- Do not clean any further.
- Do not remove the smear layer.
- If you are relying on the adhesion between the cement and the dentine to retain the crown, then **do not** cement the crown.
- The use of an adhesive cement will not compensate for a poor preparation.

Non-vital tooth

Having removed the temporary restoration and any remaining cement, condition the entire dentine, particularly in the posthole, with 10 per cent poly(acrylic acid) for 15 seconds.

- Wash thoroughly with water, then dry with alcohol followed by a gentle air stream.
- Do not dehydrate the tooth.

Placement of the restoration

- Paint the cement onto the restoration with a small stiff bristle brush.
- Paint a little cement on to the tooth as well.
- Place the restoration and apply positive pressure until the margin is fully closed. Release the pressure and maintain a dry field.
- If using a fast-setting cement, further protection is not required.
- If using a slow-setting cement, varnish liberally with the manufacturer's waterproof varnish and wait until the cement is set.
- Break off the excess cement before the cement has set too hard.

Type II.1: Restorative aesthetic cements

Dispensing

The powder/liquid ratio is important.

Capsulated

The powder/liquid ratio is already set. Follow carefully the manufacturer's directions when activating the capsule.

Hand dispensing

When dispensing the powder follow the manufacturer's directions. In particular:
● Shake the bottle
● Spoon out the powder carefully.

It is very easy to:
● Have voids in the powder and therefore underdispense
● Have spare powder on the back of the spoon or the handle and therefore overdispense.

When dispensing the liquid:
● Hold the bottle vertically upside-down
● Count the drops

● Mix half the powder at a time and complete the mix quickly. The chemical reaction begins **immediately**, and prolonged mixing will only break up the newly formed polymer chains.

Conditioning the tooth

● If there is less than 0.5 mm of dentine remaining under the floor of the cavity, place a small quantity of fast-setting calcium hydroxide over the pulp.
● To gain optimum adhesion, remove the smear layer, plaque, pellicle and any other contaminants to ensure that the dentine and enamel are in a clean condition ready for full chemical union.

Prepared cavity

Apply 10 per cent poly(acrylic acid) on a cotton pledget for 15 seconds only. Wash thoroughly with air/water spray for 20 seconds. Dry lightly. Do not dehydrate.

Erosion lesion

Clean lightly with a slurry of pumice and water. Wash thoroughly with air/water spray and dry lightly. Condition with 10 per cent poly(acrylic acid) for 15 seconds and wash again. Do not dehydrate.

Placement of the restoration

- Apply the cement to the cavity promptly. Remember, it is beginning to set already.
- Use of a syringe is desirable because positive placement will minimize porosities and voids.
- Use of a matrix is desirable but not essential. The cement will set in the presence of air but a matrix will apply pressure and adapt the material more positively to the cavity floor and walls and minimize porosities and voids.
- **Note carefully** – probably because of its chemical affinity for both tooth structure and the material of the matrix strip, the cement will not flow far in advance of the tip of the syringe. Therefore place the tip of the syringe right to the floor of the cavity, or right to the end of the tunnel. Begin to syringe and withdraw at the same time. When placing capsulated cements, it is possible to place incrementally and tamp each increment into position with a small plastic sponge.

Protection of the new restoration

- Type II.1 restorative aesthetic cements take **at least 24 hours** to achieve an acceptable degree of maturity. If aesthetics and physical properties are important, do not disturb for 24 hours.
- Approximately 4 minutes from starting to mix the cement, remove the excess cement from around the matrix, to confirm that it is set. Remove the matrix and immediately apply a liberal coat of a single component, very low-viscosity light-activated bonding resin.
- After application of the bonding resin, trim only if essential. Adjust the occlusion and remove overhangs as required.
- Apply more bond if required and activate with light. Do not disturb again for 24 hours.

Polishing

After 24 hours, polish as required, always under air/water spray.
- Trim with very fine diamonds under air/water spray
- Smooth with graded, abrasive rubber polishing points under air/water spray
- Polish with Soflex discs under air/water spray.

Maturation

For the first 6 months after placement, as chemical maturation will continue for some considerable time, be prepared to cover the restoration with a single component, very low-viscosity light-activated bonding resin if it is to be exposed to air for longer than a few minutes.

Type II.2: Restorative reinforced cements

Dispensing

The powder/liquid ratio is important.

Capsulated

The powder/liquid ratio is already set. Follow carefully the manufacturer's directions when activating the capsule.

Hand dispensing

● When dispensing the powder, follow the manufacturer's directions. In particular:
  a shake the bottle
  b spoon out the powder carefully.

It is very easy to:
  a have voids in the powder and therefore underdispense
  b have spare powder on the back of the spoon or the handle and therefore overdispense.

● When dispensing the liquid:
  a hold the bottle vertically upside-down
  b count the drops.

● Mix half the powder at a time and complete the mix quickly. The chemical reaction begins **immediately**, and prolonged mixing will only break up the newly-formed polymer chains.

Conditioning the tooth

● If there is less than 0.5 mm of dentine remaining under the floor of the cavity, place a small quantity of calcium hydroxide over the pulp.
● To gain optimum adhesion, remove the smear layer, plaque, pellicle and any other contaminants to ensure that the dentine and enamel are in a clean condition ready for full chemical union.

Prepared cavity

Apply 10 per cent poly(acrylic acid) on a cotton pledget for 15 seconds only. Wash thoroughly with air/water spray for 20 seconds. Dry lightly. Do not dehydrate.

Placement of the restoration

● Apply the cement to the cavity promptly. Remember, it is beginning to set already.
● Use of a syringe is desirable, as positive placement will minimize porosities and voids.
● Tamp into place using a small plastic sponge held in conveying tweezers.
● Use of a matrix is desirable but not essential. The cement will set in the presence of air, but a matrix will apply pressure and adapt the material more positively to the cavity floor and wall and so minimize porosities and voids.

● **Note carefully**–probably because of its chemical affinity for both tooth structure and the material of the matrix strip, the cement will not flow far in advance of the tip of the syringe. Therefore place the tip of the syringe right to the floor of the cavity, or right to the end of the tunnel. Begin to syringe and withdraw at the same time.

Protection of the new restoration

● This cement is completely resistant to water uptake 6 minutes after starting to mix. The application of a protective layer is therefore not required.
● However, if left exposed for longer than 10 minutes, for example under a rubber dam, it will dehydrate and crack. If it is necessary to leave it exposed, then it should be protected with a resin-bonding agent after polishing.

Polishing

Six minutes after starting to mix the cement, contour and polish as required – always under air/water spray.
● Trim with very fine diamonds under air/water spray
● Smooth with graded abrasive rubber polishing points under air/water spray
● Polish with Soflex discs under air/water spray.

Type III: Lining cements

Dispensing

The powder/liquid ratio is important.

Capsulated

The powder/liquid ratio is already set. Follow carefully the manufacturer's directions when activating the capsule.

Hand dispensing

- When dispensing the powder, follow the manufacturer's directions. In particular:
  a shake the bottle
  b spoon out the powder carefully.

It is very easy to:
  a have voids in the powder and therefore underdispense
  b have spare powder on the back of the spoon or the handle and therefore overdispense.

- When dispensing the liquid:
  a hold the bottle vertically upside-down
  b count the drops.

- Mix half the powder at a time and complete the mix quickly. The chemical reaction begins **immediately**, and prolonged mixing will only break up the newly-formed polymer chains.

Conditioning the tooth

- If there is less than 0.5 mm of dentine remaining under the floor of the cavity, place a small quantity of calcium hydroxide over the pulp.

Prepared cavity

Apply 10 per cent poly(acrylic acid) on a cotton pledget for 15 seconds only. Wash thoroughly with air/water spray for 20 seconds. Dry lightly. Do not dehydrate.

Erosion lesion

Clean lightly with a slurry of pumice and water. Wash thoroughly with air/water spray and dry lightly. Condition with 10 per cent poly(acrylic acid) for 15 seconds and wash again. Dry but do not dehydrate.

Placement of the cement

At the prescribed powder/liquid ratio, lining cements are very thin and flow easily. Note that they set rapidly and working time is limited. By the 'tacky' stage, no further adhesion is available. Flow into place with a small applicator, or use a syringe if placing the cement in bulk.

Protection of the cement

- The cement is set and resistant to water loss approximately 6 minutes from starting to mix, so protection is not required.
- However, if left exposed for longer than 10 minutes, it is likely to dehydrate and crack. Therefore, proceed promptly and complete the restoration.

Sandwich technique

Glass-ionomer cement is the ideal lining for all composite resin restorations. The glass-ionomer cement will provide adhesion to the dentine and will protect the dentine from the dangers inherent in the acid etch technique used for enamel adhesion.

The composite resin will provide adhesion to enamel sufficient to withstand most masticatory stress.

Selection of the glass-ionomer cement

- If optimum strength is required, choose the cement with the greatest tensile strength.
- If aesthetics is important, use Type II.1 restorative aesthetic cement.
- If radiopacity is required, use a Type II.2 reinforced cement or a Type III lining cement.
- If time is important, use a fast-setting Type II.2 reinforced cement or a Type III lining cement.
- Always use a powder/liquid ratio of 3:1 or greater.

Dispensing

The powder/liquid ratio is important.

Capsulated

- The powder/liquid ratio is already set. Follow carefully the manufacturer's directions when activating the capsule.

Hand dispensing

- When dispensing the powder follow the manufacturer's directions. In particular:
  a shake the bottle
  b spoon out the powder carefully.

  It is very easy to:
  a have voids in the powder and therefore underdispense
  b have spare powder on the back of the spoon or the handle and therefore overdispense.

- When dispensing the liquid:
  a hold the bottle vertically upside-down
  b count the drops.

- Mix half the powder at a time and complete the mix quickly. The chemical reaction begins **immediately**, and prolonged mixing will only break up the newly-formed polymer chains.

Conditioning the tooth

- If there is less than 0.5 mm of dentine remaining under the floor of the cavity, place a small quantity of calcium hydroxide over the pulp.
- To gain optimum adhesion, remove the smear layer, plaque, pellicle and any other contaminants to ensure that the dentine and enamel are in a clean condition ready for full chemical union.

Prepared cavity

- Apply 10 per cent poly(acrylic acid) on a cotton pledget for 15 seconds only. Wash thoroughly with air/water spray for 20 seconds. Dry lightly. Do not dehydrate.

Erosion lesion

- Clean lightly with a slurry of pumice and water. Wash thoroughly with air/water spray and dry lightly. Condition with 10 per cent poly(acrylic acid) and wash again. Dry but do not dehydrate.

Placement of the cement

If using a Type II.1 restorative aesthetic cement:
- Fill the cavity with the cement of choice, making sure that all the dentine is covered. Build up at least 2 mm above the gingival margin, using a matrix to support the cement if required.
- At 4 minutes from the start of mix, cover the cement with a generous layer of single component low-viscosity light-activated bonding resin and light activate. Leave undisturbed for 20 minutes. Only then proceed to place the composite resin.

If using a Type II.2 reinforced cement:
- Fill the cavity with the cement of choice, making sure that all the dentine is covered. Build up at least 2 mm above the gingival margin towards the contact area, using a matrix to support the cement if required.
- At 6 minutes from the start of mix, proceed to place the composite resin.

If using a Type III lining cement:
- Use a low powder/liquid ratio of 1.5–1.0 only if the entire cavity is surrounded by enamel strong enough to provide an enamel-bonded margin. Cover all dentinal tubules with a layer of cement at least 1 mm thick. Etching of the cement is optional under these circumstances.
- Use a high powder/liquid ratio of 3:1 or greater if any margin is in dentine or the remaining enamel is weak and friable. Overfill the cavity with the cement of choice making sure that all dentine is covered. Build up at least 2 mm above the gingival margin towards the contact area using a matrix for support.
- At 6 minutes from the start of mix, proceed to place the composite resin.

Placement of composite resin

Once the cement is set, proceed as follows:
- Trim the cement with very fine diamonds under air/water spray to final cavity outline. Remove single component low-viscosity light-activated bonding resin from areas to be etched, including the enamel. Leave the dentine covered, especially at the gingival margin.
- Bevel the enamel margins as required. Wash and dry lightly.
- Place etchant over enamel and glass-ionomer cement. After 15 seconds, wash thoroughly for 30 seconds and dry, but do not dehydrate.
- Apply resin bonding agent, blow off excess and light activate.
- Apply the composite resin and, building incrementally, complete the restoration.

Appendix

BOX E CAVITY PREPARATION INSTRUMENTS

There is a very extensive array of cutting instruments available to the profession for the preparation of a cavity and selection of the most appropriate is often difficult. The following list is presented as a starting point only in full recognition that practically all manufacturers of dental rotary cutting instruments will have their version of this list.

The main principle involved is preservation of remaining tooth structure and each of these groups of burs have been selected with this in mind.

One technique which is of great value in controlling the amount of tooth removed during cavity preparation is the use of intermediate high speed – that is 40 000–60 000 revolutions/min under air/water spray. This provides for excellent tactile sense, while at the same time allowing tooth removal at a sufficiently economical speed, particularly when preparing such fine surgical-type cavities as here advocated.

Diamond stones
a Tapered stones for entering, defining   — Intensiv 206
    Small cylinder for entering   — Horico FG 106 010
    Very fine taper for fissures   — Abrasive Technology MFS 201 MF 1

Steel burs, latch type
b Tapered fissure bur TF XC 700   — 38/010
    Small round for caries removal   — 1/011–1/016
    Long shank round   — 1/012–016 ELA
    Extra long shank   — Moller Pulp bur, Meisinger 191/120–180

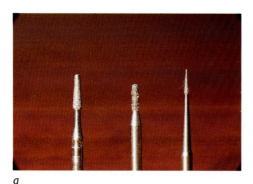

a

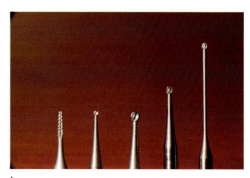

b

BOX F   SUITABLE MATRICES

Class I fissure seal
- If the matrix requires considerable strength, use Hawe Cervical Matrix no 723 and pre-shape on the tooth (see Figure 3.6).
- If the matrix requires only moderate strength, use a small section of lead foil from the back of an X-ray film. Cut it to shape and apply a very light film of low-viscosity light-activated resin or vaseline on the undersurface. It will now form to shape under finger pressure and peel readily from the set cement (see Figure 6.15).
- If the matrix does not require any strength at all, use a small piece of domestic type Glad Wrap cut to shape. Adapt with finger pressure.

Class II
- If the matrix requires considerable strength, use a conventional mild steel matrix strip either alone or in a retainer. Apply a thin coating of low viscosity light activated resin or vaseline to the inner surface before seating (see Figure 6.44).
- If the matrix requires only moderate strength, use a regular mylar strip, cut to length and wedged as required (see Figure 6.51).

Class III
- Use a regular mylar strip. Cut to length and wedge as required (see Figure 3.12).

Class V
- If the matrix requires considerable strength, preform a Hawe Cervical Matrix nos 719–723. These have already been pre-treated to allow separation from the set cement (see Figure 4.6).
- For complex two- and three-surface Class V cavities, cut heavy tin foil to shape and support as required with greenstick compound. Cut a hole in a strategic position with a round bur (1/018) and syringe the cement into place through the hole (see Figure 3.47).

BOX G   WEDGES

The purpose of a wedge is twofold. It can be used to support the gingival margin of a matrix band or to gain space between two teeth and thereby improve the strength of the contact point. It can fulfil both purposes at once.

To support the gingival margin of a matrix band

- Use a wooden wedge but take care not to distort the matrix band.
- If the matrix band is frail and likely to distort under pressure, use a small pledget of cotton wool soaked in a light-activated resin bonding agent. Place this interproximally as required and light activate. This will give sufficient support to the matrix to allow positioning of the glass-ionomer cement without displacement or production of an overhang.

- If the matrix is of heavy tin foil, support as required with greenstick compound.

To gain space between two teeth

- Plan ahead of time and place an orthodontic rubber ring one week before restoration.
- Place a wooden wedge before beginning cavity preparation. Adjust the pressure periodically prior to placing the matrix.
- If placing a posterior composite resin restoration, use a plastic light-transmitting wedge in the same manner.

Reading list

Aboush YEY, Jenkins CBG, An evaluation of the bonding of glass-ionomer restoratives to dentine and enamel, *Br Dent J* (1986) **161**: 179–184.

Aboush YEY, Jenkins CBG, The effect of poly(acrylic acid) cleanser on the adhesion of a glass polyalkenoate cement to enamel and dentine, *J Dent* (1987) **15**: 147–52.

Bass EV, Wing G, The mixing of encapsulated glass-ionomer cement restorative materials, *Aust Dent J* (1988) **33**: 243.

Blagojevic B, Mount GJ, A laboratory study of glass-ionomer cements in relation to clinical dentistry, *Aust Dent J* (1988) **33**: 320–1.

Causton BE, The physical and mechanical consequences of exposing glass-ionomer cement to water during setting, *Biomaterials* (1982) **2**: 112–4.

Causton BE, Johnson NW, Improvement of polycarboxylate adhesion to dentine by the use of a new calcifying solution, *Br Dent J* (1982) **152**: 9–11.

Cranfield M, Kuhn AT, Winter G, Factors relating to the rates of fluoride release from a glass-ionomer cement, *J Dent* (1982) **10**: 333–4.

Dahl BL, Øilo G, Retentive properties of luting cements: an in vitro investigation, *Dent Maters* (1986) **2**: 17–21.

Earl MSA, Mount GJ, Hume WR, Effect of varnishes and other surface treatments on water movement across the glass-ionomer cement surface, *Aust Dent J* (1985) **30**: 298–301.

Earl MSA, Mount GJ, Hume WR, Effect of varnishes and other surface treatments on water movement across the glass-ionomer cement surface II. *Aust Dent J* (in press).

Fitzgerald M, Heyes RJ, Heyes DR et al, An evaluation of a glass-ionomer luting agent: Bacterial leakage, *JADA* (1987) **114**: 784–6.

Forsten L, Fluoride release from a glass-ionomer cement, *Scand J Dent Res* (1977) **85**: 503–4.

Fuss J, Mount GJ, Makinson OF, The effect of etching on a number of glass-ionomer cements, *Aust Dent J* (in press).

Garcia R, Caffesse RG, Charbeneau GT, Gingival tissue response to restoration of deficient cervical contours using a glass-ionomer material — a 12 month report, *J Prosthet Dent* (1981) **46**: 393–98.

Garcia-Godoy F, The preventive glass-ionomer restoration, *Quint Int* (1986) **17**: 617–19.

Garcia-Godoy F, Marshall DM, Mount GJ, Microleakage of glass-ionomer tunnel restorations, *Am J Dent* (1988) **1**: 53–6.

Glantz P-O, Adhesion to teeth, *Int Dent J* (1977) **27**: 324–32.

Going RE, Loesche WG, Grainger DA et al, The viability of microorganisms in carious lesions five years after covering with a fissure sealant, *J Am Dent Assoc* (1978) **97**: 455–62.

Heithersay GS, Tissue responses in the rat to trichloracetic acid – an agent used in the treatment of invasive cervical resorption, *Aust Dent J* (1988) **33**: 451–61.

Heys RJ, Fitzgerald M, Heys DR et al, An evaluation of a glass-ionomer cement luting agent: pulpal histological response, *J Am Dent Assoc* (1987) **114**: 607–11.

Hicks MJ, Artificial lesion formation around glass-ionomer restorations in root surfaces: a histological study, *Gerodontics* (1986) **2**: 108–13.

Hicks MJ, Flaitz CM, Silverstone LM, Secondary caries formation in vitro around glass-ionomer restorations, *Quint Int* (1986) **17**: 527–32.

Hood JAA, Childs WA, Evans DF, Bond strengths of glass-ionomer and polycarboxylate cements to dentine, *NZ Dent J* (1981) **77**: 141–4.

Hotz PR, Experimental secondary caries around amalgam, composite, and glass-ionomer cement fillings in human teeth, *SSO* (1975) **89**: 965–7.

Hotz P, McLean JW, Sced I et al, The bonding of glass-ionomer cements to metal and tooth substrates, *Br Dent J* (1977) **142**: 41–7.

Hume WR, Mount GJ, In vitro studies on the potential for pulpal cytotoxicity of glass-ionomer cements, *J Dent Res* (1988) **67**: 915–18.

Kawahara H, Iminishi Y, Oshima H, Biological evaluation of a glass-ionomer cement, *J Dent Res* (1979) **58**: 1080–6.

Kidd EAM, Cavity sealing ability of composite and glass-ionomer cement restorations: An assessment in vitro, *Br Dent J* (1978) **144**: 139–42.

Knibbs PJ, Glass-ionomer cement: ten years of clinical use, *J Oral Rehab* (1988) **15**: 103–15.

Knibbs PJ, Plant CG, Pearson GJ, A clinical assessment of an anhydrous glass-ionomer cement, *Br Dent J* (1986) **161**: 99–103.

Knight GM, The use of adhesive materials in the conservative restoration of selected posterior teeth, *Aust Dent J* (1984) **29**: 324–7.

McComb D, Retention of castings with a glass-ionomer cement, *J Prosthet Dent* (1982) **48**: 285–8.

McComb D, Ericson D, Antimicrobial action of new proprietary lining cements, *J Dent Res* (1987) **66**: 1025–8.

McConnell RJ, Boksman L, Hunter JK et al, Effect of restorative materials on the adaptation of two bases and a dentine bonding agent to internal cavity walls, *Quint Int* (1987) **17**: 703–10.

McLean JW, Glass ionomer cements, *Br Dent J* (1988) **164**: 293–529.

McLean JW, Limitations of posterior composite resins and extending their use with glass ionomer cements, *Quint Int* (1987) **18**: 517–529.

McLean JW, A new method of bonding dental cements and porcelain to metal surfaces, *Oper Dent* (1977) **2**: 130–42.

McLean JW, Gasser O, Glass cermet cements, *Quint Int* (1985) **5**: 333–43.

McLean JW, Powis DR, Prosser HJ et al, The use of glass-ionomer cements in bonding composite resins to dentine, *Br Dent J* (1985) **158**: 410.

McLean JW, Wilson AD, The clinical development of the glass-ionomer cements I: Formulations and properties, *Aust Dent J* (1977) **22**: 31–6.

McLean JW, Wilson AD, The clinical development of the glass-ionomer cements II: Some clinical applications, *Aust Dent J* (1977) **22**: 120–7.

McLean JW, Wilson AD, The clinical development of the glass-ionomer cements III: The erosion lesion, *Aust Dent J* (1977) **22**: 190–5.

McLean JW, Wilson AD, Fissure sealing and filling with an adhesive glass-ionomer cement. *Br Dent J* (1977) **136**: 269–70.

McLean JW, Wilson AD, Prosser HJ, Development and use of water-hardening glass-ionomer luting cements, *J Pros Dent* (1984) **52**: 175–81.

Maldonado A, Swartz ML, Philips RW, An in vitro study of certain properties of a glass-ionomer cement, *J Am Dent Assoc* (1978) **96**: 785–91.

Matis BA, Cochran M, Carlton T et al, Clinical evaluation and early finishing of glass-ionomer restorative materials, *Oper Dent* (1988) **13**: 74–80.

Mount GJ, Clinical considerations in the prevention and restoration of root surface caries. *Am J Dent* (1988) **1**: 163–8.

Mount GJ, Clinical requirements for a successful 'sandwich' – dentine to glass-ionomer cement to composite resin, *Aust Dent J* (in press).

Mount GJ, Glass-ionomer cements: Clinical considerations. In: Clarke JW, ed. *Clinical Dentistry.* (Harper and Row: Philadelphia 1984) Chapter 20A.

Mount GJ, Glass ionomer cements in gerodontics. A status report for the American Journal of Dentistry, *Am J Dent* (1988) **1**: 123–8.

Mount GJ, Glass-ionomer cements – obtaining optimum aesthetic results, *Dental Outlook* (1988) **14**: 3–7.

Mount GJ, Longevity of glass ionomer cements, *J Prosthet Dent* (1986) **55**: 682–4.

Mount GJ, A method of testing the union between glass-ionomer cement and composite resin, *Aust Dent J* (1988) **33**: 462–6.

Mount GJ, Restoration with glass-ionomer cement: Requirements for clinical success, *Oper Dent* (1981) **6**: 59–65.

Mount GJ, Root surface caries – a new emphasis, *Periodontology* (1987) **8**: 31–7.

Mount GJ, Root surface caries: a recurrent dilemma, *Aust Dent J* (1986) **31**: 288–91.

Mount GJ, The tensile strength of the union between various glass-ionomer cements and various composite resins, *Aust Dent J* (in press).

Mount GJ, The use of glass-ionomer cement in clinical practice, *Dental Outlook* (1982) **8**: 37–44.

Mount GJ, The wettability of bonding resins used in the composite resin/glass-ionomer 'sandwich' technique, *Aust Dent J* (1989) **34**: 32–5.

Mount GJ, Makinson OF, Clinical characteristics of a glass-ionomer cement, *Br Dent J* (1978) **145**: 67–71.

Mount GJ, Makinson OF, Glass-ionomer restorative cements: Clinical implications of the setting reaction, *Oper Dent* (1982) **7**: 134–141.

Ngo H, Earl MSA, Mount GJ, Glass-ionomer cements: a 12 month evaluation, *J Prosthet Dent* (1986) **55**: 203–5.

Øilo G, Evje DM, Film thickness of dental luting cements, *Dent Maters* (1986) **2**: 85–9.

Pameijer CH, Segal E, Richardson J, Pulpal response to a glass-ionomer cement in primates, *J Prosthet Dent* (1981) **46**: 36–40.

Pameijer CH, Stanley HR, Bio-compatibility of a glass-ionomer luting agent in primates. Part 1, *Am J Dent* (1988) **1**: 71–6.

Phillips RW, The restoration of eroded cervical areas, *CDS Review* (1980) **73**: 31–2.

Phillips RW, Swartz ML, Lund MS et al, In vivo disintegration of luting cements, *JADA* (1987) **114**: 489–92.

Powis, DR, Folleras T, Merson SA et al, Improved adhesion of a glass-ionomer cement to dentine and enamel, *J Dent Res* (1982) **61**: 1416–22.

Prodger TE, Symons M, Aspa adhesion study, *Br Dent J* (1977) **143**: 266–77.

Prosser HJ, Characterisation of glass-ionomer cements. 7: The physical properties of current materials, *J Dent* (1984) **12**: 231–40.

Prosser HJ, Powis DR, Wilson AD, Glass-ionomer cements of improved flexural strength, *J Dent Res* (1986) **65**: 146–8.

Reisbick MH, Working qualities of glass-ionomer cement, *J Prosthet Dent* (1981) **46**: 525–30.

Skorland KK, Bacterial accumulation on silicate and composite materials, *J Biol Buccale* (1976) **4**: 315–22.

Smith DC, Ruse ND, Acidity of glass-ionomer cements during setting and its relation to pulp sensitivity, *JADA* (1986) **112**: 654–7.

Sneed WD, Luper SW, Sheer bond strength of a composite resin to an etched glass-ionomer, *Dent Mater* (1985) **1**: 127–8.

Stokes AN, Proportioning and temperature effects on the manipulation of glass ionomer cements, *J Dent Res* (1980) **59** (spec. issue Pt 1): 1782.

Swartz ML, Phillips RW, Clark HE, Long term fluoride release from certain cements [Abstract], *J Dent Res* (1984) **63**: 158–60.

Thornton JB, Retief DM, Bradley EL, Fluoride release from and tensile bond strength of Ketac Fil and Ketac Silver to enamel and dentine, *Dent Maters* (1986) **2**: 241–5.

Tobias RS, Brown RM, Plant CG et al, Pulpal response to a glass-ionomer cement, *Br Dent J* (1978) **144**: 345–50.

Tviet AB, Gjerdet NR, Fluoride release from a fluoride-containing amalgam, a glass-ionomer cement and a silicate cement, *J Oral Rehabil* (1981) **8**: 237–41.

Tyas MJ, Clinical performance of adhesive restorative materials for cervical abrasion lesions, *J Dent Res* (1983) **62**: 646, Abstr. 512.

Vougiouklakis G, Smith DC, Lipton S, Evaluation of the bonding of cervical restorative materials, *J Oral Rehabil* (1982) **9**: 231–51.

Walls AWG, Glass polyalkenoate (glass-ionomer) cement: a review, *J Dent* (1986) **14**: 231–46.

Warren JA, Soderholm K-JM, Bonding amalgam to glass-ionomer with polyacrylic acid, *Dent Maters* (1988) **4**: 191–6.

Welbury RR, Factors affecting the bond strength of composite resin to etched glass-ionomer cement, *J Dent* (1988) **16**: 188–93.

Wilson AD, Crisp S, Lewis BG et al, Experimental luting agents based on the glass-ionomer cements, *Br Dent J* (1977) **142**: 117–22.

Wilson AD, McLean JW, *Glass-ionomer cement.* (Quintessence: London 1988).

Wong TCC, Bryant RW, Glass-ionomer cements: Dispensing and strength, *Aust Dent J* (1985) **30**: 336–40.

Wong TCC, Bryant RW, Glass-ionomer cements: Some factors in film thickness, *Aust Dent J* (1986) 81–5.

Index